The Whole Man Program

Reinvigorating Your Body, Mind, and Spirit after 40

Jed Diamond

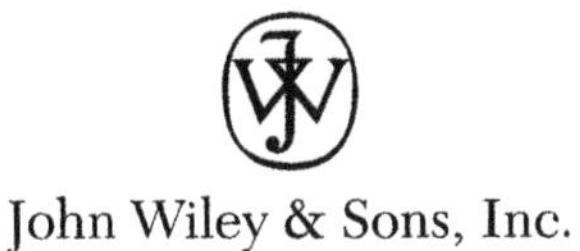

John Wiley & Sons, Inc.

Also by Jed Diamond

Surviving Male Menopause: A Guide for Women and Men
Male Menopause
The Warrior's Journey Home: Healing Men, Healing the Planet
Looking for Love in All the Wrong Places
Inside Out: Becoming My Own Man

Published by John Wiley & Sons, Inc., New York
Published simultaneously in Canada

The author gratefully acknowledges permission from the following sources to include material in this book:
From *Worry* by Edward M. Hallowell, copyright © 1997 by Edward M. Hallowell, M.D. Used by permission of Pantheon Books, a division of Random House, Inc.
From *The Wonder of Boys* by Michael Gurian, published by Tarcher/Putnam, a division of Penguin Putnam, Inc. Used by permission.
10 Reasons to Exercise by Ken Goldberg, M.D., used by permission.
From *Stiffed: The Betrayal of the American Man,* copyright © 1999 by Susan Faludi, reprinted by permission of HarperCollins Publishers, Inc.
From *The Testosterone Revolution,* copyright by Malcolm Carruthers, M.D., reprinted by permission of HarperCollins Publishers, Inc.
Material on Tom Sipes' vision quest by permission of Tom Sipes.

Library of Congress Cataloging-in-Publication Data

Diamond, Jed, date.
The whole man program : reinvigorating your body, mind, and spirit after 40 / Jed Diamond.
p. cm.
Includes bibliographical references and index.
ISBN: 0-471-26756-2
1. Middle aged men—Health and hygiene. 2. Health. 3. Longevity. 4. Sexuality. 5. Physical fitness. I. Title.

RA777.8 .D53 2002
613'.0434—dc21 2001046959

10 9 8 7 6 5 4 3 2 1

This book is dedicated to all of the men and women
who have shared their stories with me over the last 37 years.
It is through their struggles and dedication
to men's health that this book is possible.

Every serious thinker must ask and answer three fundamental questions:

(1) What is wrong with us? With men? Women? Society? What is the nature of our alienation? Our dis-ease?
(2) What would we be like if we were whole? Healed? Actualized? If our potentiality was fulfilled?
(3) How do we move from our condition of brokenness to wholeness? What are the means of healing?

—Paul Tillich

CONTENTS

ACKNOWLEDGMENTS

I WANT TO THANK my wife, Carlin, for her commitment to having a healthy husband in her life. She has been a wonderful role model for health and a committed partner.

My children Jemal, Angela, Aaron, Evan, and Dane keep me oriented toward the future and continually challenge me to practice what I preach.

Nancy Ellis continues to be a magnificent agent, always going the extra mile to ensure that my literary health continues to deepen over the years.

Tom Miller, my editor at John Wiley & Sons, has helped make this book a much better one than it would have been without his suggestions, support, and challenge.

I want to thank my colleagues in the field of men's health, particularly Dr. Will Courtenay, Dr. Malcolm Carruthers, Dr. Clement Williams, Dr. Ken Goldberg, Dr. Warren Farrell, John Lee, Erin Pizzey, David Shackleton, Jean Bonhomme, Ron Henry, Steven Svoboda, Marilyn Milos, Tracie Snitker, Bert Hoff, Gordon Clay, and Jim Bracewell.

My assistant, Norman Roscoe, has kept all my various tasks coordinated and has been a tremendous help in putting the final touches on the book.

I want to thank the men in my group for their personal support, for being models of the kind of men whose health improves as they age, and for their lifelong commitment to stay together.

I want to give special thanks to all the men and women who have opened their hearts and shared their stories with me. Your courage has inspired me many times when my own courage had failed. Your commitment to health makes the world a better place for us all to live.

INTRODUCTION

I AM A 58-YEAR-OLD married man. I have five children and, as of the writing of this book, eight grandchildren. I have been interested in men's health since I was 6 years old, when my father became seriously ill.

I was a biology major in college and went into medical school after I graduated. My interest in the psychosocial aspects of health quickly deepened and I soon left the study of medicine and enrolled in the School of Social Work at the University of California at Berkeley.

The women's movement was beginning to have an impact on the wider society and a number of women's health clinics were being started. There was a recognition that women's health needs were different than men's and required a gender-specific approach to healing.

At that time many believed that all health care was geared toward the needs of men—that everything, other than the few clinics for women, was family and general health care. Following that reasoning there would be no need for a specific focus on men's health. I didn't believe that was true then and I don't believe it is true now.

I have written this book to show the importance of a specific health program for men and to give men specific guidance in using the program to stay healthy as we age. My 37 years of experience in the health field has convinced me that it is just as important that men have a health program that speaks to our needs as it is that women have a program that focuses on their unique health concerns.

Some people are afraid that an approach to health that takes into account the differences between men and women would lead toward inequality and poorer care for one sex. I don't believe that needs to be the case. Acknowledging the differences in our health needs, as well as the similarities, can go a long way toward ensuring that men and women are as healthy as it is possible for us to be.

Most people would agree that men and women are different. There are obvious differences in our bodies. But the differences go beyond our anatomy. We now know that men's and women's brains are different, both in structure and in operation. We have different reactions to many medications. We deal with stress in different ways. Our emotional vulnerabilities differ. We contract disease and die at different rates. It's time we acknowledged the differences and developed programs to meet the specific needs of men as well as women.

This approach is becoming accepted globally. "While a gender-specific approach is often used to identify persistent inequalities in the status of women," says a recent report from the World Health Organization, "the specific situation of men, particularly older men, also requires investigation and further studies, especially with regard to the determinants of health."

—ɷ—

I also wrote this book because there are significant differences between the health issues that younger men experience and those that we experience as we get older. For instance, prostate infections are quite common in younger men. Prostate enlargement is often present as we age. Violence is the cause of death for many young men. The lack of intimacy and love is the cause of death for many older men.

In our younger years we often took our health for granted. We didn't learn all we could because we didn't think we needed to do anything specific to stay healthy. As we get older it is clear that we need more information, and we need the support to act on that information.

The third reason I wrote this book is that my experience convinced me that we needed an integrative approach to healing that took into account all aspects of men's health. It isn't enough to focus on getting men to go to the doctor more often. In fact, men's reluctance to go to doctors may be because we know that seeing a doctor is not the most important aspect of health.

We need to focus on nutrition, hormones, physical activity, feelings and emotions, our career and calling, understanding women, and how to develop intimacy. We need to learn how support from other men can be lifesaving. And we need to learn how all these aspects of health can work together.

Staying healthy can be so much fun. Health is too important to be taken seriously. We need to add more joy into our health practices. In my younger years I thought fun was eating poorly, drinking too much, and watching TV sports on weekends. Now I'm more inclined to enjoy great food, drink moderate quantities of excellent wine, and play sports on the weekends. There are so many ways to enjoy staying healthy as we age, and I want to share them with you.

—ɷ—

I write the kinds of books I would like to read. When talking about health, I want good factual information. I also want it clear and personal. I distrust going to a doctor who gives me advice on health but appears unhealthy himself. I want to know about him and if he practices what he preaches. In this book I'll tell you about my own experiences, what I do to stay healthy, and what I've learned working with men over the last 37 years.

Although this is a men's health book, it isn't just for men. I know you are interested in information that can help your husband, brother, father, and son. Women are often in the position of being the family health expert. I know there are many things you want to know about a man's unique health needs.

One of the greatest tragedies of life is that so many of you spend many years alone after the premature death of your spouse or must watch as a once vital man deteriorates and goes downhill as he ages. That doesn't need to be the case. This book is here to help you help him.

—~—

This is a wonderful time to be alive. For the first time in human history we are able to experience the full potential of our genetically programmed life span. Many men and women are now living well past 100 years, and their numbers are expected to rise dramatically over the next 25 years. Not only are we learning how to add years to our life, but how to add life to our years. Nearly every day there are new breakthroughs in science and medicine that offer promise for a longer and better future.

The real challenge will be for us to learn how we can best use these added years. There are so many opportunities to make use of our gifts and talents. I invite you to join me in exploring this future together. We are all pioneers in a new world in which we can all live long and well.

—~—

I'm pleased you are reading *The Whole Man Program.* It has been a joy to research and write, and I hope you will find it a joy to read. I want to tell you a little about what you will find in the book and some ideas about how to move through the book to get the most out of it.

In Part I we will look at the positive potential for living long and well in the second half of life. You will learn about the research on men who have lived healthy and productive lives and are still going strong past their hundredth birthday. We will see what these men can teach us about life. I will share my own health journey and the progress and direction of the new men's health movement. You will learn about andropause, or male menopause, and how this critical life stage can determine our future health and well being.

In Part II we explore the problem that men face today. You will learn why we currently die sooner and live sicker than women, the reasons we don't take better care of ourselves, and about the male shame that often keeps us stuck in unhealthy patterns.

In Part III you will be given the first section of the Men Alive Program for Total Health. You will learn the secrets of how to eat well so you never develop a potbelly and lower your risk of ever suffering a heart attack. You will learn about male hormones and testosterone replacement therapy. You will find out what kind of physical activity is best for you and learn how to have fun exercising for life.

In Part IV you will explore the inner world of feelings and emotions and receive guidance to keep your emotional life happy and healthy. You will learn the difference between your "career" and your "calling" and how to live your calling in the second half of your life.

In Part V you will be given the third part of the Men Alive Program, which focuses on the vital importance of intimacy and love in keeping us vital and healthy as we age. You will get a glimpse inside a men's group and find out why its members feel it may be the key factor contributing to their physical, emotional, and spiritual health.

You will learn about the phenomenon of gender shifting and find out why men become more gentle, sensitive, and caring as we age. You will be introduced to the archetypal Woman and feel how she influences all our relationships. Finally, you will learn the most valuable, and perhaps the most difficult, health practice: how to have an intimate partnership that stays sexy and alive throughout the ages.

In Part VI you will be invited to take the Eight-Week Men's Health Challenge to put into practice what you have learned and begin a health journey that will last the rest of your life.

—w—

This is an action-oriented book. You don't need to wait until the end of the book to put something you learn into practice. I hope you will stop reading at many points in the book and take time out to *do something.* Believe me, if you want your health to improve, you need to *act* on what you learn.

If you read something that sounds good, try it out. See how it might work in your life. You'll never know until you try. I've also included a number of plainly marked Action Options. These offer you specific suggestions for putting what you are learning into practice.

At the end of the book I have included a bibliography of readings that will allow you to delve more deeply into the subject of men's health. There is also a resource section that will allow you to use the Internet to keep up on the latest information in the emerging field of gender medicine.

There are a number of ways you can use this book, and you'll probably find ways I haven't even thought of.

1. You can start at the beginning and read on through to the end, doing the Action Options as they come up.
2. You can go to specific chapters that interest you right now and take action in those areas that concern you the most.
3. You can think of the first four parts of the book as a four-month program and do a part each month.

If you decide to complete the Eight-Week Men's Health Challenge it will help if you've read the whole book, and you will need to be familiar with the chapters in the program section of the book.

I expect that many of you will work with this book through the years. You will want to pick it up again and again to review certain sections that will relate to health issues you are dealing with at that time.

I hope you will stay in touch with me and let me know what is working for you. I would also like to know about new discoveries you find and new resources you think would be helpful to others. One of the main goals of the book is to let men know we are not alone and that we can help each other to stay healthy and live well.

The best way to reach me is by e-mail: Jed@menalive.com. I also have an online newsletter and information through my web site: http://www.menalive.com.

PART I

Men's Health over 40

CHAPTER 1

How Men Can Live Long and Well

> The truth is, part of me is every age. I'm a three-year-old, I'm a five-year-old. I've been through all of them, and I know what it's like. I delight in being a child when it's appropriate to be a child. I delight in being a wise old man when it's appropriate to be a wise old man. Think of all I can be! I am every age, up to my own.
>
> —Mitch Albom, *Tuesdays with Morrie*

"I PLAN TO LIVE to 130," said Daniel, a good-looking man in his early 50s. He had come for health counseling to achieve his goal. I asked him how he came up with 130 as the age he aspired to. He told me he had read my book, *Male Menopause,* and was encouraged to find that more and more people were expected to live past 100. "Since some people today live to be 120," Daniel said with a smile, "and we continue to learn more and more about extending the life span, it seems reasonable that I ought to be able to make it to 130 and be healthy to boot. Besides, I kind of like the idea of living to the retirement age of 65, then having a second full life of 65 years ahead of me."

Certainly Daniel is not alone in his desire. Long life has been a dream that humans have always sought. For most of our 3 million year history, human beings died once their reproductive peak had passed. As late as 1910, the average life expectancy at birth in the United States was 50 years—slightly lower for males, a bit higher for females.

Yet, for the first time in human history, we now have a chance to see the full extent of the human life cycle. Recent research on aging and longevity has led some in the field to predict that we are just beginning to find out the potential for human life. No one wants to live to be 100 or more and be sick and debilitated. But if we could live long and also be healthy, that is a future that most people would be interested in seeing. The idea that the older we get, the sicker we get, and the more likely we are to die, may not be true. According to research reported in the University of California, Berkeley *Wellness Newsletter,* "If you make it to age 80, you have a better chance of living to 100 than you had at age 70."

For many of us, our view of an "old man" was a guy in a hospital bed with tubes running in and out of his body. At best it was an old codger with white hair doddering down the walk at the old folks' home on his way to the cafeteria for his evening meal of cooked carrots and peas. With this view of aging, most of us would rather follow the old dictum, "Live fast. Die young."

Most of us are raised with the belief that we must compromise our desires of what the good life is like as we get older. Some of us think we can be financially secure in our old age, but that we have to drive ourselves at work and pay the price of our health. Others think we can be healthy, but that it means we have to live life in the slow lane and give up financial security as we get older.

I believe we can have it all. Why not be rich *and* healthy rather than sick and poor? But we need a clear vision of how good life can be in our 50s, 60s, 70s, 80s, and beyond. We need to be aware of the obstacles to having a long, healthy, and prosperous life. Finally, we need to have the courage to overcome the obstacles and go after the life we all want.

How Men Can Thrive Despite Obstacles: My Father's Story

My father was a man who had to overcome many obstacles in order to live long and well. Like many men in midlife, he struggled with feelings of failure. When he was unable to make a living at his chosen profession, writing and acting, he slipped farther and farther into despair. No one knew how depressed he was because he rarely appeared to be sad. He was more often irritable and angry. He would leave the house and be away for long periods of time. When he was at home, everything seemed to bother him. He refused to get help when it was offered, claiming he could handle things by himself.

When I was five, he tried to kill himself. After his suicide attempt, he was committed to the state mental hospital. With the primitive approaches used to treat mental illness at the time, he regressed even further. My uncle would take me each Sunday for a visit, but it became evident that my father was slipping farther and farther away and soon didn't even recognize me. I was confused and frightened. After two years in the hospital, the doctors told my mother that he would never leave alive. They felt he would either succumb to the depression and kill himself or regress so completely he could end up in a permanently psychotic state.

In fact, my father did neither. After spending eight years in the hospital, one day he escaped. He hitchhiked to Los Angeles, took on a new name, and at the age of 51 began a new life. He always lived in fear that someone would recognize him and send him back to the hospital, which he referred to as "the concentration camp."

That may have been one of the reasons that he became a puppeteer. With the attention on the puppets, there was much less focus on him. He earned money by doing temp work and by passing the hat when he did his impromptu shows. In the past, his life was focused on trying to get good acting jobs and getting his books and plays published. He always worried that he wasn't making enough money. Now his life was focused on making children happy and getting adults to think. He would tell me in later years, "Money is never a problem. There's always enough for what is truly important."

I remember him from my childhood as being angry—angry at agents, publishers, the government, the guy who cut him off in traffic, and my mother when she tried to be helpful. Now he seemed to have found some kind of inner peace. I asked him once what had changed. "I'm just happy to be alive and free," he told me. "Each day is a gift and I feel so full of gratitude for all that I have."

We had gotten to be close friends in his later years. He had fought and conquered many of his inner demons. Mentally, he was sharp as a tack. He never kept an appointment book and he never forgot one of our luncheon dates. He also remembered the baseball scores and what the Giants needed to do to get into first place. Physically, he was strong. His handshake at 85 was as strong as mine at 45, and I worked out three times a week. He walked every day, taking his puppets all over San Francisco. When he was 80 he decided to quit smoking, saying he wanted to stay as healthy as he could.

Later that same year he decided to become a vegetarian. "It's much healthier," he told me. "And besides, we shouldn't be killing animals like that."

He had many friends all over the city. Many people remembered him from when their parents took them to see one of his puppet shows. Now they brought their own children to see "the puppet man." Even living on his small Social Security check, he said he always felt rich. He never passed someone in need on the street without giving that person a dollar or two. "When the great puppet man in the sky calls me," he said, "I'm not going to need my money, so I might as well give it to someone who can use it now."

Although he rarely got paid, he always had a job. He considered it his duty to put on puppet shows at many of the San Francisco convalescent hospitals as well as for those who waited each day in the food lines. Even when he was sick, which he rarely was, he would get up each day, dress, and go out to do his work. "People expect me," he would say. "I don't want to let anyone down." He wasn't religious, although he was proud of his Jewish heritage. He was deeply spiritual and committed to social justice.

It was appropriate that the last walk we took was to attend the opening of the new San Francisco public library. He said he wanted to see it completed and to bring some flowers to honor all the people who had helped in bringing it into being. He was proud that a new library was being built close to his neighborhood.

It was a long walk from his small room to the library, and we proceeded slowly. He didn't talk much. He held my arm with one hand, carried his bouquet of flowers in the other. When we arrived he sat on a bench and asked me to deliver the flowers. When I returned he seemed deep in thought. He clasped my knee in a grip that was as solid as a vise, smiled, and said, "It's been a good day. It's time to go now."

I thought he meant time to return to his room. Two days later he was taken to the hospital with a slight case of pneumonia. Two days after that he died. It had been a good day and a good life for a man for whom midlife was just the beginning. Einstein once said that one should strive "not to be a man of success, but a man of value." In taking that last walk with my father, I came to understand what he meant.

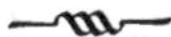

I am fortunate to have other exceptional models for how men can continue growing psychologically and spiritually as well as maintaining their health as they age. I picture my Uncle Harry at 95 still singing the songs that he had written over the last 80 years, the ones that had gotten him into the Songwriter's Hall of Fame: "Sail Along Silvery Moon," "Miss You," "It's a Lonesome Old Town," and hundreds of others. He never wanted to rest on his success. He was out plugging his music to each new generation of singers.

I smile when I think of my teacher in graduate school, Sidney, who is still living well at 87. He still exercises every day, plays the violin, and has weekend excursions with his lady friend. His joy for life is infectious. He is truly a man who is living long and well.

Rather than being the long-lived exceptions, it may turn out that men like these will be the average. If we take good care of ourselves, we may be able to live even longer and maintain good health as we go.

These are the findings of the New England Centenarian Study, based at Harvard Medical School and Beth Israel Deaconess Medical Center in Boston. Thomas Perls, M.D., was the director of the study. He hopes his findings can help us all live long and well. After studying people who live to be 100, Perls was surprised to find how healthy they were: "It's really amazing to think about an additional forty years of good health beyond a person's sixties."

The study found that most of us are living way below our potential for a long and healthy life. They found that the average person is born with a set of genes that would allow us to live to 85 years of age and maybe longer. Those of us who take appropriate preventive steps may add as many as 10 quality years to that. If we fail to heed the messages of preventive medicine we will likely subtract substantial years from our lives.

Many of us think of old age as living long in spite of our illnesses, going downhill the longer we are alive. It's why most of us would rather live hard and die young. But the research in the New England Centenarian Study indicates that people live to 100 not by living in spite of disease, but by avoiding or delaying it as long as possible. They have replaced the saying "The older you get, the sicker you get," with the more accurate observation "The older you get, the healthier you've been."

Expanding Your Vision of Health and Well-Being

At our clinic we believe that health is not just the absence of illness, but is a positive state of well-being. In order to be healthy we need to avoid the habits that work against us. But we also need to have a positive vision of how we would like things to be. Here's a quiz that will help you explore your own hopes and desires.

Your View of Health

1. How long would you like to live if you could maintain your health throughout your life?

2. Think of older people you know who are in good health. What are the things about them that are healthy?
3. What does good health mean to you?

Physical Well-Being

4. Do you have any physical symptoms that concern you?
5. Do you feel fit?
6. Do you do physical activities that will prevent disease?
7. Do you neglect your health until there is a problem?
8. Do you tend to work at a sedentary job and get most of your exercise as a "weekend warrior"?
9. Do you get some combination of aerobic, resistance, and stretching exercises in the course of a week?

Emotional Well-Being

10. Do you feel real joy and delight in your life?
11. Do you often feel frustrated, down, or worried?
12. How easy is it for you to express a range of emotions: anger, hurt, fear, guilt, and love?
13. Do you tend to blame others or yourself when things don't go right, or do you accept yourself and others as OK even when mistakes are made?

Family Health Risks

14. What health problems did members of your family of origin have?
15. Did you grow up in a home where there was violence, drug or alcohol abuse, mental illness, or other family stress?
16. Did you grow up in a family with a mom and a dad who had trouble showing love to each other or their children?
17. What have you done to reduce the risks of repeating these problems?

Food Practices

18. How knowledgeable are you about healthy eating?
19. How well do you put into practice what you know?
20. Are you ever compulsive about what you eat or how you eat?
21. Do you feel "hooked" on certain foods?
22. Do you drink as much water as you should (8 glasses a day)?

Intimate Partnerships

23. Are you married or in a long-term, intimate relationship?

24. How happy are you in your relationship?
25. Do you feel understood, respected, and loved?
26. Are you and your partner friends as well as lovers?
27. Can you be yourself, with your excesses and deficits, and still be accepted?
28. Is there room in your relationship for closeness and freedom?
29. Do you renew the relationship so that it can grow over time?

Family, Friends, and Community

30. How do you feel about the members of your family?
31. Are there old hurts from the past that haven't healed?
32. Do you find time to be together?
33. Do you have friends that you can be open and honest with?
34. Have you ever been in a men's group?
35. Would you consider joining one?
36. Do you recognize the importance of friendships?
37. Do you nurture old friendships and develop new ones?
38. Do you feel connected to your community?
39. Do you feel you have something vital to contribute?

Stress Management

40. What are the major sources of stress in your life?
41. Do you recognize that a good deal of our stress comes from our perceptions of events, not the events themselves?
42. What strategies do you use to handle stress?
43. Does stress ever cause you to feel irritable or detached?
44. Do you keep stress bottled up inside?
45. How easy is it for you to relax?
46. Where do you turn for support or comfort?

Irritability and Anger

47. Do you find that you are often irritated by life's challenges?
48. Are family, friends, or colleagues often a source of frustration to you?
49. Do you have periodic blowups during which you raise your voice?
50. Do you ever feel intense anger when you are driving?
51. Are you like a pressure cooker building up steam inside?
52. Do you ever turn your anger outward and hurt those you love?
53. Do you turn your anger inward and cause yourself physical pain or emotional turmoil?

Mind-Altering Substances

54. Do you smoke cigarettes or chew tobacco?
55. Do you ever drink too much alcohol?
56. Does your use of caffeine from soft drinks, tea, or coffee cause you to become jittery or keep you awake at night?
57. Do you feel groggy until you get going in the morning?
58. Do you need a cup of coffee to get you going?
59. Do you have trouble taking medications as prescribed?
60. Are there other drugs that have caused you trouble in your life?
61. Do you have trouble stopping using substances even when you have decided it is necessary?

Spiritual Life Purpose

62. Does your life have meaning?
63. Do you feel you have something special to contribute to the world?
64. Do you feel needed by your family?
65. What do you know that if generally practiced would make the world a better place?
66. Does your work have a purpose beyond bringing home a paycheck?
67. Do you feel you are expressing who you really are?
68. Do you feel appreciated for who you are and what you give?

Joy in Life

69. Can you still be inspired by beauty and wonder?
70. Can you still be silly and playful?
71. What things do you truly enjoy?
72. Do you take the time to have fun?
73. Who do you know who is really fun loving?
74. What could you do to allow that quality to express itself in you?
75. How often do you just let yourself go and enjoy life with reckless abandon?

Unique Gifts

76. Do you have things that you'd like to share with others?
77. Are there things you've learned that you'd like to teach?
78. Do you have opportunities to express love and give to others?
79. Do you honor and appreciate yourself?
80. Do you recognize that with all your excesses and deficits you are a great man?

—∾—

How honest have you been in answering these questions? We all want to look good, even to ourselves. There is always a tendency to answer the way we'd like it to be, rather than the way it really is. We all do it. It's important to recognize the tendency, so we don't avoid dealing with important areas of our lives that need attention.

I hope you can see that health is more than simply the absence of disease. Health is a by-product of living a full and joyful life. We all get in ruts and get stuck. Sometimes we are stuck for a long time. Do you recognize any areas of your life that are keeping you from full enjoyment? Have you recognized any old patterns that you have gotten caught in, even though they aren't working? Are there positive aspects of your life you would like to enhance? Are you ready to begin changing some of these destructive patterns and deepen the positive aspects?

A Program for Change

How many times have we wanted to do something that we thought would make us healthier? "I know I need to lose some weight," we tell ourselves. "This time I'm going to stop smoking," we say as we crush a cigarette out in the ashtray. Sometimes our resolutions made in the heat of the moment disappear with the evening mists. Other times we actually start to make a change but it doesn't last, or we are successful for a while and then fall back into old patterns.

If we've lived 40 or 50 years or more, we have made many attempts to improve our health. Most seem to have failed. It's no wonder we get discouraged and try to convince ourselves that it's OK to be overweight, underexercised, overstressed, and depressed.

The real problem is that most of us have never learned how change works and how to create lasting, healthy, joyful, changes in our lives. The changes that are easy, we do without much effort. How difficult is it to change your brand of toothpaste? How much thought do you need to put into getting the oil changed in your car?

The changes that most of us make (and break) are much more difficult to achieve. We usually have conflicting desires and resistance about the change even if these desires and resistance are not apparent. Think about losing weight, or exercising more, or reducing stress, or taking more time to relax. These changes don't come easy, and we shouldn't feel discouraged if change is difficult.

We need to understand that change occurs as a result of specific steps that if followed, greatly increase our chances of success.

The Twelve Steps for Successful Change

1. Feel discomfort about how things are in your life.

The first step in changing something is recognizing that something is not right about how things are at present. It may be a vague sense: "I just don't feel like my old self." Or it can be more specific: "I feel too fat."

2. Think about how you would like things to be.

We need a vision of the future, something to look forward to if we are to change. At this point the desire can be vague or specific: "I want to feel the kind of energy I once had." "I want to fit into my pants without feeling stuffed."

3. Get specific about what you would like to change.

Now we need to be specific about what we want to change. It's important that we be as detailed as we can about what we'd like. Don't limit yourself by the past. This is a new day and a new program. Go for what you really want. List some specific things you want to change. For example:

- I want to lose weight.
- I want to feel less pain in my joints when I wake up in the morning.
- I want more time for myself.
- I want more intimacy between my wife and myself.

Even if you aren't ready to make changes in all these areas of your life, it is good to feel the freedom of having them written down, so you can see what you really want. Many of us won't even let ourselves know the truth of our own desires.

4. Prioritize your desires.

Although changing one area of your life may bring about changes in other areas, it is important to prioritize the changes you want to make. In our enthusiasm to make a new beginning in living more healthy lives, we may try to do everything at once. We need to think about what's most important. Here is my personal list, in order of priority, for the coming year:

- I will lose weight.
- I will improve my flexibility.
- I will reduce my stress level.
- I will improve my sex life.
- I will have more time and money for travel.

5. Pick a desire and examine the benefits as well as the resistance and drawbacks to taking action.

This is a critical step that most of us overlook. We naively assume that all our desires are "obviously" beneficial. Clearly losing weight, improving flexibility, reducing stress levels, improving one's sex life, and having more money to travel will all be good things. But everything in life is a trade-off and the failure to recognize the pros and cons of possible actions is often the reason that we fail to meet our goals.

My primary desire is to lose weight. Here are the benefits I feel I will gain:

- I will have more energy.
- My clothes will fit better.
- I will like how I look.
- I will be healthier.
- I will feel sexier.
- I will be quicker and play better racquetball.
- My wife will like my appearance.
- I will be a good role model for other men my age.
- I will feel good that I could accomplish a difficult task.

Thinking of benefits is usually easy. What is more difficult is thinking of the drawbacks or resistance we have. If there were no drawbacks, any change, like losing weight, would be easy.

Here are the drawbacks I think I would experience:

- I would have to give up eating foods that I enjoy like cakes, cheese, pizza, candy, bread, jellies, and jams.
- I wouldn't feel free to eat whatever I want at parties or potluck dinners.
- I would have to exert my willpower and say no.
- I would have to eat less.
- I might be unsuccessful and feel like I was a failure.

All of us have our own set of perceived benefits and drawbacks. There are no rights or wrongs. Our reasons for wanting to change or not wanting to change may seem silly or trivial. If they are real to us, they are important.

6. Make the decision to change.

It's only after looking honestly at our benefits and drawbacks to change that we can make a real decision. It isn't just adding up the number of things on each side of the list, either. Some listings carry a greater weight than others. It's OK at this point to say no. It may well be that I "should" lose weight, that others "know" it would be good for me, that it is the "right" thing to do. The truth may be that in the scale of my life at this time, the benefits to losing weight just don't outweigh the drawbacks.

However, if we can honestly say that the scales tip, no matter how slightly, in the direction of losing weight, I am ready to make a decision. I state it with all my commitment and resolve. I will lose weight.

7. Decide on a goal.

This is another area where many of us fail. Making a decision to lose weight isn't enough. Changes need to be quantifiable and time limited. Another way to say that is by asking myself how I will know when I get there. Losing weight is great, but how much do I commit to losing and over what time frame? Whatever your commitment, you need to be able to know when you have crossed the finish line. My personal goal is to lose 20 pounds in six months.

For me, losing 20 pounds over that time is a realistic goal that I can achieve without going on a crash diet, which would only backfire. Many of us make changes in the short run, only to have them reversed in the long run. I want to lose weight and keep it off.

8. Have an action plan.

For change to occur we need a plan of action. Leaving things to chance is a setup for failure. Here we need to break our long-term goal into small steps and create a plan for moving ahead. In my case, to lose 20 pounds in six months I will need to lose just over 3 pounds a month. Here is what I will do to lose those 3 pounds every month:

- Play racquetball three times a week.
- Do yoga or other flexibility exercise at least once a week.
- Do strength exercises three times a week.
- Eat fruits, vegetables, and whole grains every day.
- Avoid cakes, candies, cheeses, bread, butter, jellies, and jam.

9. Anticipate obstacles and come up with answers.

We often make plans to change while pretending there are no obstacles, and then we are surprised when we run into them. It helps to anticipate what is likely to get in our way so we can plan in advance what we will need to get past them.

Obstacle: Get hungry for something quick when I'm on the road.
Answer: Take healthy foods with me to snack on.
Obstacle: Get hungry for "something good" before I go to bed.
Answer: Eat well earlier. Drink herbal tea to relax.
Obstacle: Forget the benefits of losing weight and get off my plan.
Answer: Read the benefits to losing weight and recommit one day at a time.

10. Seek support.

I often think, "No one can help me but myself. If I need to make a change I have to do it on my own."

The older I get the more I realize how much support I need. It isn't usually easy for us to reach out and ask for help, but the rewards are great. Not only do the people we reach out to help us achieve our goals, but they connect us to others in a positive way.

Here's what I intend to do to get support:

- Ask my wife to encourage and appreciate my changes.
- Call on men in my group to check in with me and hold me accountable for what I have committed myself to do.
- Appreciate myself for my efforts and be gentle with myself if I should slip.
- Picture myself being the weight I want to be.

11. Monitor your changes.

It's always a good idea to monitor our changes. Not only does it give us a reference point to see how we are doing, but success will encourage a desire for more success.

I will weigh myself every day and record my progress in a notebook. Since weight varies a good deal on a daily basis, I will do weekly averages to monitor my changes over time.

If some aspect of my program isn't working, I will talk to one of my health-conscious friends about helping me modify the program, rather than abandoning it.

12. Maintain your program.

I just talked to a friend last night who is considerably overweight. He and his brother both wanted to lose weight. Last New Year's Day they made a bet on who would lose the most weight in six months. My friend said at the end of six months he looked and felt great. He had lost 58 pounds. His brother had lost 59.5 pounds. Though he lost the bet, he was happy with his weight loss.

The problem, as you might guess, was that he had no program for maintaining his progress, so as soon as the bet was over, he went back to his old pattern of eating poorly and exercising rarely. He also said, "The diet just about killed me. I hated it."

My plan is to do a program that I will enjoy and can maintain long after the six months are up.

These are the twelve steps to lasting change. They have worked for me many times and have worked for hundreds of men we have seen at our health clinic. They will work for you, too. Real change, though, is never easy. It takes courage and commitment. If you're simply interested in going through the motions of getting healthier, this program isn't for you. If you're doing this for someone else, you're likely to go through the motions, but not really achieve your goals: "See, honey, I really am trying to get healthier."

This is a program for those of you who are truly "sick and tired of being sick and tired," a popular phrase in addiction recovery. Unhealthy living *is* an addiction. It is just as destructive as shooting heroin or smoking crack cocaine. Healthy living is freedom. It allows us be the men we have always wanted to be. It allows us to live life with passion, joy, and courage. I invite you to join me. The journey will be exciting and rewarding.

My Personal Health Program

1. I am primarily a vegetarian (though I eat fresh fish occasionally) and eat lots of vegetables, fruits, and grains. As I say in chapter 7, I continually work keeping my diet healthy. It isn't easy for me.
2. I take a high potency multivitamin and mineral supplement three times a day.
3. I play racquetball two or three times a week. I practice flamenco dancing twice a week and walk as much as I can. I'm planning to add some yoga practice to increase my flexibility.

4. I take two medications, under the supervision of a physician, to treat a mood disorder that I have had all my life and runs in my family.

5. I have been taking a testosterone gel, under the supervision of a medical specialist, to treat my testosterone deficiency.

6. I take an herbal formula that includes saw palmetto and pygeum to prevent and treat prostate enlargement.

7. I have regular medical checkups once a year and see my doctor as needed. I get regular PSA (prostrate specific antigen) blood tests to check for prostate health as well as the DRE (digital rectal exam—which is a very minor discomfort and not nearly as uncomfortable as all the male joking would imply). I also had my first sigmoidoscopy, where they stick a tube up your butt to check for colon cancer. Again, no picnic, but way better than my fears.

8. I am in two men's support groups. One has been meeting for over 21 years and meets four or five times a year. The other one meets every other week. Both give me a deep sense of connection with other men.

9. I spend a good deal of time in person and by phone with our children and grandchildren. My wife, Carlin, and I also plan regular time together. We still have a Wednesday night "date night," which we have maintained throughout our marriage. We have both been married twice before, and we recognize the importance of nurturing our relationship.

10. We live in a beautiful spot, surrounded by trees, which is very quiet and serene. We are a half mile from our nearest neighbor and a half hour from the wonderful town of Willits, California, a three-and-one-half-hour drive from San Francisco.

11. I love quiet time alone. I try and walk in the woods at least two or three times a week. Every night before I go to bed, I spend a half hour alone reading.

12. I have a passion for my work, which feels more like play than "work," and love the balance between writing, seeing clients, teaching, consulting, and training.

CHAPTER 2

My Own Health Journey and the New Men's Health Movement

> Few things get a person more interested in being healthy than a big bout of being sick. I define "health" as a happy, vibrant life, doing the most with what you have, with delight.
>
> —Patch Adams, M.D.

The Journey Begins

It was cold that late November day in 1969. My wife and I were tired of the looks we received from friends as they looked at her bulging belly. Their eyes would lift and the question was obvious. "Not yet, huh?" My wife's eyes replied with a mixture of anxiety and anger: "No, not yet, as you can see. But it better be soon."

I was a month shy of my 26th birthday. My wife was 22. It was our first child and we were both ready for the birth. The childbirth classes had ended. We had practiced our breathing, packed her bags, and some pictures to focus her attention, and received the well wishes of friends. All we needed now was for the baby to decide the time was right to come into the world.

I admit, I had agreed to join the birthing classes and to be with my wife through the labor because it seemed to be the right thing to do. Most of our friends who were pregnant were doing it. My wife wanted me to be there. I wanted to support her. My terror was that I would pass out in the delivery room and have to be carried out before they could attend to the birth. I had never done well with blood. It was one of the reasons I had dropped out of medical school.

The contractions began in the afternoon and we dutifully timed them. When we were sure the birth was imminent, we called the hospital. I tried to remain calm, but I was at the edge of panic. My wife seemed to be taking it in stride. When we got settled into her room, the nurse checked her and told us that we had a long way to go.

I helped her pace her breathing and wiped her forehead. I fed her ice chips and rubbed her neck and shoulders. There was a young girl who was sharing the room, and though she was on the other side, it was clear that she was alone and very frightened. I offered some words of encouragement and was glad I was with my wife to give her support.

As the hours progressed and we wondered if it would go on forever, I thought of what the Kaiser Hospital doctor had told us. Whether the father would be allowed in the delivery room would be up to the doctor who was on duty at the time of the birth. When I began the process, I found myself hoping that we'd get a traditional doctor who would want me to wait outside. That way I could save face with my wife: "Darn, I wanted to be with you all the way, but the doctor wouldn't let me."

But as time went on and I felt more connected to my wife and our soon-to-be-born baby, my desires began to shift. I wanted to be there for the whole show. Leaving began to feel like abandoning my wife and child. It also felt like I would be missing the last act of a play that had begun nine months ago. "I might be scared," I thought, "but I'm not going to let myself pass out. I want to be there."

When the contractions were the most intense and her breathing was coming in short gasps, the nurses said it was time to move into the delivery room. As they transferred my wife from the bed to the gurney to wheel her in, the nurse informed me that the doctor asked that I now wait in the waiting room.

A wave of relief washed over me as I hugged my wife and squeezed her hand. "Maybe it's for the best," I thought. "They don't need a frightened father to contend with." I began my long walk down the hallway leading away from the delivery room toward the waiting room to join the other expectant fathers.

I was surprised to find that I didn't feel frightened. I felt frustrated. As I got ready to push through the exit doors leading to the waiting room, I found I couldn't make myself go through. Something drew me back, some force beyond reason. I turned around and walked back up the hallway and into the delivery room. I took my place at the head of the table and gave my wife a kiss on the forehead. There was no question of my leaving if asked. I was here to stay. My place was with my wife and our soon-to-be-born son.

Minutes later, amid tears of pain and delight my son, Jemal, was born. His cord was cut and the doctor handed him to me.

At the moment in which I looked into his beautiful face I made a vow in answer to his call for me. I told him I would do everything I could to be a father who was totally involved in his life. I told him that I would be there for him now and forever. I told him I would never wait in life's waiting rooms even if society told me that's where a father belonged. I told him I would be a more involved father than my father had been able to be. I told him I would do everything I could to create a world where men remained healthy throughout their lives in body, mind, and spirit. In those few moments we crafted a bond that I know will last a lifetime.

The Growth of My Involvement in the Men's Health Movement

In those early years I felt a great deal of support from my wife, her women friends, and from the women's movement in trying to be a different kind of man than my father had been. I realized I wanted a better world, not only for my son, but also for myself.

In 1976, when Jemal was 7 and I was 33, I read a book that helped me understand the pressures my father had faced and what men continued to face every day as they tried hard to be the manly men that society demanded. In *The Hazards of Being Male: Surviving the Myth of Masculine Privilege,* psychologist Dr. Herb Goldberg focused attention on the destructive aspects of the male role. "The male has paid a heavy price for his masculine 'privilege' and power," says Goldberg. "He is out of touch with his emotions and his body. He is playing by the rules of the male game plan and with lemming-like purpose he is destroying himself—emotionally, psychologically and physically."

During that time I also read *The Liberated Man* by Warren Farrell. Farrell shared my hope and the hope of many men to break down the traditional roles that had kept both men and women in relationships that limited their full potential. Farrell wrote: "Men's involvement in breaking out of the strait jacket of sex roles is essential because of the way it confines men at the same time it confines women."

I experienced, firsthand, the way these roles helped destroy the lives of my father and mother. My father was a gentle man who was lousy at competing in the work world. He was much better at being an artist and a writer. My mother loved to work and was a natural leader. Though she loved being with me, she craved other stimulation. She became depressed trying to support my father in work he hated while keeping her own ambitions under wraps.

"As soon as men define themselves as the only ones capable of handling certain situations, of being aggressive, of earning the most money, " says Farrell, "then a woman who is equally capable in these areas becomes a threat to his very self-definition." It was my desire to understand what limited my parents and to break out of the restrictions that limited them that led me to writing.

In 1983, my own book on men's health, *Inside Out: Becoming My Own Man,* was published. In it I described the underlying beliefs that had influenced me and seemed to have influenced most men I knew. Even though I could see how destructive these rules of life were, I didn't fully appreciate how difficult it was to change them. Twenty years after I first wrote them, I still struggle trying to keep them from destroying my health, my peace of mind, and my life.

I called them *The Commandments That Move Me:*

- I can never be weak.
- If I have a weak moment I must hide it from everyone, including myself.
- I must never fail at anything.
- To fail is to lose my sense of self. To fail my family is to lose my reason for living.
- I must work to support my family whatever the cost to myself. To ever lose a job is to feel shame at the core of my being.
- I cannot express emotions, particularly love, fear, or sadness. Anger is sometimes acceptable if directed at other men.
- I must not cry, complain, or ask for help.
- I must never be uncertain or ambivalent. If I'm not always sure of myself, I must act that way.
- I must not be dependent or act like I need someone.
- Disrespect is my greatest fear. I'm afraid I might kill or die rather than live a life where I felt disrespected.
- I must ignore my own health. "Real men" are indestructible.
- If I'm sick or injured I must "play hurt." To slow down to take care of myself is unmanly and a source of shame.

It was important for me to recognize that these commandments had become so much a part of my life that they had become invisible. They operated below my awareness, yet influenced me every day. They were developed early on in my life. I remember at age five being told that big boys don't cry. At seven, when I was being beaten and tormented by an older girl, I was told a boy must never hit a girl. In junior high, when I had surgery on my leg, I was told to be strong, not to complain. On the high school basketball team, I learned to play hurt and ignore pain.

ACTION

Develop New Guidance for Life

Look over my list of "commandments." Pick one that particularly fits the way you were raised. Give yourself a more realistic statement to live by now. For instance, you may have picked "I can never be weak." A more realistic statement might be "I'm a human being and there will be times when I feel weak." Practice this new statement at least twice a day for the next week.

When we are young our youthful minds and bodies could take a good deal of mistreatment before they let us down. Many of us are now paying the price as we get older. What are some of your concerns now about your health?

These books and a few others on men's health made some impact at the time but did not bring about the kind of social change that was true of the women's health movement. "There are several reasons why the men's health movement has made comparatively little progress," says Dr. Will Courtenay, founder and director of Men's Health Consulting. "The women's health movement was successful, in part, because it was linked with a larger social movement—one that addressed the many inequalities that women experience in this country. But there is another reason why progress has been slower for the men's health movement. That reason is because most of us men have been working in relative isolation from one another."

This is beginning to change. In 1990 a number of men recognized that men's health was something that all aspects of the men's movement could agree upon and started the Men's Health Network. The goals were simple, yet profound:

1. To save men's lives by reducing the premature mortality of men and boys.

2. To increase the physical and mental health of men so that we can live fuller and happier lives.

3. To significantly reduce the cycles of violence and addiction that afflict so many men.

Based in Washington, D.C., this group was instrumental in bringing national attention to men's health issues and for getting Congress to proclaim the week before Father's Day as Men's Health Week. Members also staff a men's health line offering timely information on a variety of men's health issues.

About the time the Men's Health Network was getting started a new magazine was born. Called simply *Men's Health,* the magazine's editors felt that men were beginning to take notice of their health and well-being. For those that argue that men are not interested in their health, it should be noted that *Men's Health* now has a circulation of 1.6 million readers, more than *Rolling Stone, GQ, Esquire,* or *Men's Journal.* More than 80 percent of the readership is male.

The revitalization of the men's health movement is being driven by the reality that the population is aging. As we men reach our mid-30s, 40s, and 50s we begin to experience the body changes and life changes that make us ready to focus on our health and well-being. In our teens and 20s we felt we were invincible and didn't concern ourselves with our health. In our late 20s and early 30s, we were so busy we didn't take time to pay attention to our health. In our late 30s and 40s, we begin to slow down, either by design or necessity, and are forced, sometimes kicking and screaming, to recognize that our bodies, minds, and spirits are not made out of steel and will give us trouble if we don't care for them.

This change of consciousness is not just going on in the United States, but is occurring throughout the world. In 1998 the World Health Organization proposed and organized the first World Congress on the Aging Male, and the International Society for the Study of the Aging Male was started that same year. Conferences are taking place every two years in various parts of the world.

In the United States the importance of men's health is becoming recognized by Congress. On July 27, 2000, Senator Strom Thurmond joined Representative Randy "Duke" Cunningham in introducing a bill that will establish an Office of Men's Health (OMH) within the Department of Health and Human Services. "As one of the thousands of men who have been saved from prostate cancer by a simple PSA test, I understand the importance of regular health screenings for men," said Representative Cunningham.

A longtime champion of men's health issues, Thurmond at age 97 is living proof that our nation's predominately silent men's health crisis can be put to an end. Senator Thurmond also worked to pass the bill establishing the National Men's Health Week in 1994, which is celebrated annually during the week leading up to and including Father's Day. Whether you agree with his politics, Thurmond has been on the job longer than any senator in history. He knows something about men's health that could help us all.

The men's health movement is now coming of age. Both males and females want to know how men can remain healthy—physically, emotionally, sexually, and spiritually. But it will be a new kind of health movement, not just an extension of what has been in the past. One of the statistics that is often offered as an indication of men's resistance to taking care of themselves is that men make 150 million fewer visits to the doctor each year than do women. But another interpretation might be that men don't believe that going to the doctor is the best way to improve their health.

Men's Health: A New System for a New Millennium

Men may well be right in their belief that availing themselves of the health care system is not the best way to stay healthy. In a striking report published by the Robert Wood Johnson Foundation it was demonstrated that health status is influenced much more by our behaviors than by our going to doctors.

In fact, in looking at what contributes to the state of our health the report found that only 10 percent of our health status results from access to health care, 20 percent is a result of environmental influences, 20 percent is a result of genetics, and a whopping 50 percent is a result of our lifestyle and behaviors. According to William Reynolds Archer, M.D., Texas commissioner of health, one of the most important contributors to our health or sickness is our social connectedness. "Loneliness, isolation and depression are the real underlying causes of much of our ill health as we move into the 21st century," says Dr. Reynolds. "The real solutions will involve developing a clear purpose for our lives which connects us to our families, neighborhoods, and communities."

I'm not suggesting that we stop going to doctors or that we abandon the medical system. Rather, I'm suggesting two things: First, that we recognize a good part of getting healthy and staying healthy can be achieved without ever going to see a doctor. Such things as stopping cigarette smoking, cutting back or stopping alcohol use, eating healthier, getting more exercise, reducing stress in our lives, spending more time with friends, getting more sleep, and taking more vacations can all be effective ways of staying healthy. Second, we need to make our contacts with the health care system more productive and valuable so that men will want to go to the doctor more often.

Our Clinic

At our clinic we reach out to men in a number of ways. We have office hours in the evenings and on weekends so that men can come in without missing work. We do health screenings in the workplace so that men can have needed tests done without having to take extra time off. Perhaps most importantly, we spend time getting to know the men who come to our clinic so it feels like they are coming to talk to a trusted friend rather than an impersonal technician.

Each man I see at the clinic receives two one-hour evaluation sessions. The first question I ask is "What would you like in coming to see me today?" I want to help men begin thinking about solutions, rather than problems. I believe this is a good approach for people, but it is particularly important for men. When we go to the doctor, the first question we usually hear is some variation of "What's your problem today?"

Most of us are less interested in talking about problems than in getting to solutions. Once you know we are action oriented, you are more likely to open up about other areas of your life. Many of us hate going to doctors because we feel that we are treated like body parts rather than as whole human beings. We treat our cars in a more holistic way than we treat ourselves. Few of us would feel good about a mechanic that fixed the carburetor but completely ignored the tires, the belts, or the oil levels.

I want to know more about *you.* If you've come in hoping for help with your back pain, I may suggest acupuncture to deal with the pain, herbs to deal with the inflammation, and exercises to help keep your body flexible. But I may also ask you about your levels of stress at work. I'll want to know how you and your wife are getting along and what kinds of financial pressures you are experiencing. I'll see how much weight you carry around and what kind of exercise you are getting. I'll talk to you about what you put into your body, including your food preferences and habits, how much alcohol you drink, what you smoke, how much caffeine you use. I'll ask about your friendships and how much time you spend with friends. I'll ask about your community involvement and what you give back for all you've received. I'll even ask about your spiritual life and your sense of being connected to some presence or power beyond yourself.

We often complain that even when men come to see a doctor they are mostly silent and refuse to open up about what is really troubling them. But is this the fault of the patient, or of the way our health care system forces everyone to work quickly and impersonally? When the focus is on health care as a business, it is easy for even well-meaning and caring health care workers to fall into the trap of getting the person in and out as quickly as possible so that another paying customer can come through the door.

Yet it doesn't have to be that way. "Patients unabashedly offer their trust, love, respect, and much more to a physician who projects a caring, joyous demeanor," says Dr. Patch Adams. So why isn't there more joy in our doctors' offices? The first cause is poor communication. The joys of relationships are lost if a physician can spend only short periods of time with patients; gone is the thrill of intimacy. If physicians could really delve into their patients' lives and take time to understand the whole person, all-important lifestyle issues could be addressed.

Most doctors will tell you they don't have enough time to spend with their patients. "I'd like to be able to spend more time. I know I can't do the kind of job that is needed with a five- to seven-minute rushed interview, but there's only so much of me to go around. What do you expect me to do? I'm already stressed to the max."

Under the old system where the doctor was seen as the only point of real help that the patient could expect to get, patient needs didn't have a chance of being met. The old refrain "I'm sorry, you'll have to ask the doctor" reminded everyone that only the doctor had the answers and the other "health care professionals" were there to support the all-knowing doctor.

But again that is beginning to change. We are recognizing that total health requires a multimodality approach that focuses on many areas, including physical, nutritional, emotional, interpersonal, sexual, hormonal, economic, and spiritual health. We are also finding that there are many healing modalities beside what traditional Western medicine has to offer. Among the healing therapies now available are acupuncture, aromatherapy, bodywork, Chinese herbal medicine, chiropractic, homeopathy, massage, meditation, nutritional therapies, relationship therapy, Western herbal medicine, and yoga.

At our clinic we offer many of these modalities, and we also consider that everyone on the staff—including those at the front desk, the billing staff, the nurses, the nurse practitioners, the social workers, the psychologists, the massage therapists, and the acupuncturists—contribute equally to a patient's health care. We also include the patient themselves, family, friends, and other people taking their turn in the waiting room as part of the health team.

I will often stop and listen to the interchange between the women at the front desk and the patient when he checks in. The staff usually asks how the patient is feeling, how his kids are, what's happening out at the mill. I can see the patient relax. Whatever he came here to see the doctor about is already starting to be healed through caring interactions with the staff.

Though the doctor may only be able to spend 10 or 15 minutes with the patient, as a clinical social worker, I can spend 30 to 60 minutes with him, and I may see him every week as opposed to a doctor visit every six months. As do all members of the staff, I have my own area of specialty, but because we interact with each other, we all learn a good deal about a broad range of healing practices.

Men's Health Support Groups

We also encourage and support our patients talking to each other. I conduct a men's health support group once a week. One of the clients, a 45-year-old security guard named Dennis, recently joined the group. He had some interesting things to say about how he came to the clinic and what his initial response was.

> I'll tell you the truth. I didn't want to be here. I resisted all the way. The only reason I came was because my wife said she'd leave me if I didn't get some help with my anger and take better care of myself physically.
>
> I knew this was a different kind of place when I first arrived and saw you throwing a football around with a bunch of kids in the parking lot. You waved and asked me if I wanted to play. What kind of a health clinic is this, I wondered? When I got inside the surprise continued. There were the usual toys in the corner for kids and women's magazines on the wall. But there were also magazines that I would enjoy reading. I saw Men's Health, Esquire, and Harvard Men's Health Watch.
>
> There were pamphlets about reducing stress, fathering, and financial planning. There were posters inside talked about prostate cancer protection, avoiding erectile dysfunction, living to be 100. I hadn't realized until I got here all the clinics I had ever attended were focused on the needs of women and children. No wonder I didn't feel comfortable. I still don't relish coming to a doctor, but when I need care you can bet I'll come. For now, I'm glad I've got the group to help me deal with my the causes of my anger.

I purposely start the group about 15 minutes late because I know a great deal of health care occurs as the men hang out and talk to each other before the formal part of the session occurs. I see them leaning against their trucks, animatedly exchanging views and news about our town and their involvement in it. We also end about 15 minutes early since I found out that the guys usually walk out together and talk about what went on in the group. I found that they often open up and talk more freely after the session is over. I often walk out with them, and in the more informal atmosphere of the parking lot the real healing takes place.

Things are indeed changing in the world of health.

In the next chapter we will look at a time of life that we all must go through. Some call it the midlife passage; others call it menopause or andropause. Whatever we call it, we must recognize that it is a crucial transition time that will help determine how we live the second half of our lives.

CHAPTER 3

Andropause—Male Menopause

> Can you imagine me with a woman old enough to be my wife? No, really. I'm serious. Can you imagine me walking into Spago with a 70-year-old woman? Forget it. I don't have that spirit. My girlfriend is 25 years old—perfect.
>
> —Tony Curtis, age 70

THE YEAR I WAS BORN, my father was 38 years old. He was going through what was then called a midlife crisis. What I remember about those early years were his frequent absences. He always seemed restless and would take weekend trips looking for work that often lasted for weeks. His career as an actor and writer was stalled, and my mother had gone to work to bring in more money. I could tell it was a source of shame for him that he couldn't get work that would allow him to be a man in his own eyes and in the eyes of his wife.

During one of his trips I overheard a conversation between my mother and her women friends that had a profound impact on my life. They were talking about their husbands, all of whom didn't seem to be living up to some measure of success that would make them acceptable in the eyes of their wives. I heard my mother say, "He's either gone when I need him or he's always underfoot. Of the two I'd rather he were gone. When he's here he's always moping around the house."

What I remember more than the words was the tone in the women's voices. It was a mixture of pity, contempt, and ridicule. As a four year-old I made vow to myself: I would never let women talk about me like they had talked about my father. I would rather die first. That oath translated in later years into a commitment that I would never be out of work, that I would do anything to be sure my family had money, and that I would in fact be willing to die rather than break my commitment.

In later years I realized that my father was operating with similar beliefs. When I was nearly 40 I came across a journal that he had left. I found a number of entries that were dated around the time he was going through his own male menopause passage, though there was no name for it at the time.

> June 4th:
> Your flesh crawls, your scalp wrinkles when you look around and see good writers, established writers, writers with credits a block long, unable to sell, unable to find work, yes, it's enough to make anyone, blanch, turn pale and sicken.

> August 15th:
> Faster, faster, faster, I walk. I plug away looking for work, anything to support my family. I try, try, try, try, try. I always try and never stop.

> November 8th:
> A hundred failures, an endless number of failures, until now, my confidence, my hope, my belief in myself, has run completely out. Middle aged, I stand and gaze ahead, numb, confused, and desperately worried. All around me I see the young in spirit, the young in heart, with ten times my confidence, twice my youth, ten times my fervor, twice my education. I see them all, a whole army of them, battering at the same doors I'm battering, trying in the same field I'm trying. Yes, on a Sunday morning in early November, my hope and my life stream are both running desperately low, so low, so stagnant, that I hold my breath in fear, believing that the dark, blank curtain is about to descend.

As a midlife man myself I can feel my father's pain as his self-esteem slowly eroded away, the fear and frustration of trying to support a family took its toll, and the tide of shame began to envelope him.

Six days after his November 8 entry, my father tried to kill himself. Though he survived physically, emotionally he was never again the same.

Over the last 35 years I've treated more and more men who are facing stresses similar to those my father experienced. The economic conditions and social dislocations that contributed to his feelings of shame and hopelessness continue to weigh heavily on men today. I've come to see that this transition period—which I call male menopause, or andropause—is critical to men's survival and how they will live the second half of their lives.

Luckily my father survived, but his depression deepened and he was eventually hospitalized. He and my mother divorced. In some ways my whole life has been dedicated to understanding why he left and why so many other men leave at this time of life—through divorce, disease, despair, or death.

My father loved baseball and used it as a metaphor for life. He said that you have to keep coming up to the plate no matter how many times you strike out and that you only win by getting around all three bases and making it home.

If second base is midlife, I believe we are losing our males at three places along the base paths of life. Too many young men never make it to first. What they see early on in their lives convinces them that there is little hope. Their philosophy seems to be "live fast, die young." They end up in prison, on drugs, or dead on the streets.

Other men are afraid of getting old. They become obsessed with youth and beauty. These are the guys who won't accept that aging is a necessary reality and want to stay "forever young." They think they will find happiness by leaving their partners for someone younger and prettier. They are afraid to make the turn toward home; instead, they run past second base and end up alone in left field.

A third group makes the turn at second, but sees the later years as times of increasing loss. They believe all their worthwhile years are in the past. They expect to deteriorate, to get old and sick. I see them going past third and ending up dead in the dugout.

The key to success, as my father said, was to make it around all three bases and get home safely. Perhaps then one can become a coach and help others make the journey successfully.

Male menopause (andropause) is the stage of life that prepares a man to move from the first half to the second. Just as adolescence is a transition period and ideally prepares a child to become an adult, male menopause helps men to move from first adulthood to second adulthood. I call this transition period midlife adolescence; author Gail Sheehy calls it "middlescence." For those who have the courage to make the journey, the second half can be even more fulfilling than the first.

However, I see too many men who get lost at this stage of life. Women have a specific biological marker that tells them they are moving into a new stage of life. For men, the change is less clear and often more troublesome. We are really 20 years farther behind in our study of andropause than we are in the study of menopause. Medical experts are just now beginning to recognize the reality of male menopause.

What Are the Medical Experts Saying About Male Menopause (Andropause)?

- Marc Blackman, M.D., chief of endocrinology and metabolism at Johns Hopkins Bayview Medical Center, says, "The male menopause is a real phenomenon and it does similar things to men as menopause does to women, although less commonly and to a lesser extent."
- Aubrey M. Hill, M.D., author of *Viropause/Andropause: The Male Menopause,* says, "My experience has now convinced me that most men undergo what could be called male menopause and that many men suffer acutely and needlessly."
- Malcolm Carruthers, M.D., author of *Maximising Manhood,* says, "Andropause is a critical health concern for men and the women who love them. Its often-insidious onset can be at anytime from the age of 30 onwards, though typically it is in the fifties. One of the reasons it's often missed is that it is usually more gradual in onset than the menopause in the female, although it is more severe in its long-term consequences. It is a crisis of vitality just as much as virility, even though its most obvious sign is loss both of interest in sex and of erectile power."
- The majority of participants at the second World Congress on the Aging Male, which was held in Geneva, Switzerland, in February 2000, believed that andropause was an important life transition for men. I was one of over 800 researchers, scientists, and clinicians representing over 50 countries worldwide attending the congress. When asked whether they thought there was a significant hormonal aspect to andropause, over 80 percent said they did and would prescribe testosterone or other hormones for men who needed them.
- Jonathan V. Wright, M.D., and Lane Lenard, Ph.D., authors of *Maximize Your Vitality and Potency,* say, "Although the idea has been around in one form or other for thousands of years, until *very* recently the existence of a hormonally driven male menopause analogous to

that experienced by women was widely denied by the forces that rule mainstream medicine. Officially in this country, it still does not exist, although incontrovertible scientific evidence to the contrary has finally begun a slow shift in attitude."

Male Menopause or Andropause: What's in a Name?

The term "male menopause" is obviously inaccurate. The term "menopause," introduced by French doctors in the 1870s, combines two Greek words—*menses* ("periods") and *pausis* ("stop"). Men don't have a period, so they don't stop having one. I chose to use male menopause when I wrote two books on the subject because I found there were so many similarities between what women and men experience. The major difference is that men can continue having children following this change of life, where women's reproductive lives end.

A number of names have been used to describe this important life transition: male menopause, andropause, viropause, the male climacteric, penopause, and andropenia. All indicate that there is a change or ending that occurs in male functioning. Increasingly I am using the term "andropause" (*andro,* from the Greek word meaning "male," and *pausis,* from the Greek word meaning "stop").

The name indicates there is an ending of a certain aspect of maleness, which I'll describe in more detail later, and the beginning of a new stage. It also focuses on the fact that there is a drop in male hormones, particularly the androgens (*andro,* "male," and *gen,* "to give"), like testosterone at this time of life.

What Are the Signs We Are Moving into Andropause?

The most common signs of andropause include the following:

1. Reduced libido or sex drive
2. Reduced potency or ability to obtain and maintain an erection
3. Fatigue or loss of vitality
4. Irritability and grumpiness
5. Aches, pains, and stiffness
6. Depression that often manifests as anger or boredom

7. Night sweats or "hot flashes"
8. Dryness and thinning of the skin
9. Restlessness and a longing to break free
10. Weight gain, especially acquiring a potbelly.

At What Age Does Andropause Begin?

Andropause generally begins between the ages of 40 and 55. However, for some men it can begin as early as 30 or as late as 65. I recommend that men begin having their levels of testosterone checked in their 30s, before they experience any signs. It is more important to know how our testosterone levels change through the years than to know our absolute level.

How Long Does Andropause Last?

Andropause generally takes 5 to 15 years to complete. How long it takes depends on many factors. Remember, this is not simply a psychological shift from one stage of life to another, but involves all seven dimensions: hormonal, physical, psychological, interpersonal, social, sexual, and spiritual. We don't go from adolescence to adulthood overnight. The change from first adulthood to second adulthood generally takes as long or longer than moving through puberty.

It also depends on how tightly we cling to first adulthood. Many men have a fanatical desire to stay forever young. They associate becoming older with becoming frail, sexless, and lifeless. The more we cling to the past the longer it takes to embrace the future. The journey is inevitable. We can no more resist andropause than we can resist puberty. We can fight it, but we can't avoid it. Inevitably we must move through it to the other side.

How Many Men Are Going through the Andropause Passage?

- In the United States there are 25,172,000 men between the ages of 40 and 55 who are now going through the andropause passage.
- In less than 25 years, by 2020, the number of men in the United States going through the andropause passage will grow to approximately 57,500,000.
- Worldwide there are approximately 408 million men between the ages of 40 and 55 who are going through the andropause passage.

- By the year 2020 the number will grow worldwide to approximately 690 million men.

Do Men Experience Hormonal Cycles?

Lowered levels of hormones at midlife are central to the changes associated with andropause. Testosterone is one of the significant hormones that decreases as men age, but there are testosterone cycles that occur throughout a man's life.

We now know that men, like women, experience complex hormonal rhythms that affect their sexuality, mood, and temperament. For instance, researchers have found five different testosterone cycles in men:

- Rhythmic fluctuations three to four times an hour. (Could this account for research that shows that men think about sex every 15 minutes?)
- Daily changes with testosterone higher in the morning and lower in the afternoon.
- Fluctuations throughout the year with levels higher in October and lower in April.
- Decreasing levels associated with andropause that occur as men get older.
- Monthly fluctuations that are rhythmic, but different for each man.

"The morning highs, daily fluctuations, and seasonal cycles whip men around," says Dr. Theresa L. Crenshaw, author of *The Alchemy of Love and Lust.* "Think about the moment-to-moment impact of testosterone levels firing and spiking all over the place during the day, and what this must be doing to a man's temperament."

Is Andropause the Result of Men's Loss of Testosterone as We Age?

Some clinicians and researchers believe that andropause is primarily the result of our loss of testosterone. It's clear to me that it is much more than that. Andropause is a multidimensional change of life with hormonal, physical, psychological, interpersonal, social, sexual, and spiritual aspects. All aspects are equally important and all must be understood and treated. They are all present with men during this period of time, though they may not all be of equal intensity or equally obvious.

Andropause and Adolescence: Similar Life Stages?

I often describe andropause as adolescence the second time around or as puberty in reverse. During puberty, male hormones, such as testosterone, surge mightily. We've all experienced the signs. As Michael Gurian, author of *The Wonder of Boys,* says, "When a boy hits puberty, the influence of testosterone on the brain increases manifold. His testosterone level itself will increase in quantities ten to twenty times more than girls. His genitals will increase to eight times their previous size. His body will process anywhere between five to seven surges of testosterone per day. You can expect him to masturbate continually, bump into things a lot, be moody and aggressive, require a great deal of sleep, lose his temper, want sex as soon as he gets up the emotional guts to propose to a partner, and have a massive sexual fantasy life."

Do any of these changes sound familiar to you? Think about what we're seeing at this time of life:

- Mood swings
- Hormonal shifts
- Confusion about sexuality
- Desire to break away from family and at the same time clinging tightly to family for support
- Obsession with the latest toys and gadgets
- Need for intimacy and fears of getting close
- Physical changes in the body
- Questions about identity and direction in life

I think we all recognize these signs. But are we looking at a 15-year-old or a 50-year-old? Retitle Gurian's book in your mind and call it *The Wonder of Midlife Men* and think about our dropping testosterone. Do any of the changes feel familiar?

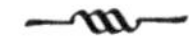

ACTION OPTION

Compare Adolescence and Midlife

Get out a piece of paper and write down the changes you remember from adolescence. Be as specific as you can. Detail a few memories from that time to illustrate each change you remember experiencing. Take another piece of paper and write down the changes you notice (or noticed) that you experienced when you were between 40 and 55. Again draw on specific memories to illustrate each change. Put a check by the changes on your two lists that are similar.

—ᴥ—

The similarity between adolescence and andropause is one of the reasons that midlife parents have such a difficult time dealing with their teenage kids. They are both working through the same issues. When Dad freaks out thinking about his daughter's emerging sexuality, it is often because he is also dealing with changes in his own sexuality. When a father has difficulty setting reasonable limits on his son's behavior, it is often because he is having trouble setting limits for himself.

Why Haven't We Heard More about Andropause?

Men respond to their life changes in a way that reflects our culturally acquired self-image. We often deny them. For us, going through this time of life is frightening. We may already feel like we are losing it, that our manhood is deserting us. Admitting that these changes may be hormonal as much as psychological may raise more fears.

This denial extends to the largely male scientific and medical communities and accounts for why it has taken so long to study andropause in more depth. We, who are out of touch with our body rhythms, afraid that "cycles" are feminine and hence to be avoided at all costs, are unlikely to be aware of the whisperings within until they become shouting.

What Is the Purpose of Andropause?

The purpose of andropause is to signal the end of the first part of a man's life and prepare him for the second half. Male menopause is not the beginning of the end, as many fear, but the end of the beginning. It is the passage to the most passionate, powerful, productive, and purposeful time of a man's life.

I often think of life as climbing up a mountain. At some point we reach our highest level and begin coming down the other side. It's not surprising that we are frightened of the changes associated with the downside of the mountain. For most of human history we died when we reached the bottom. As late as the turn of the century the average life span was only 47 years. Those of us who reach 50 can expect to live another 30 years. Many of us will live to be 100 or more.

There is a second mountain for us to climb, one that allows us to be more relaxed and less driven, more playful and less serious, more accepting and less demanding of ourselves and others. However, in order to get to this second mountain, we must go through the andropause valley. We can't jump from peak to peak. But in order to be successful on this second mountain we have to recognize that it is quite different from the first.

Many of us are slow to recognize the benefits of life on the second mountain. When confronted with our changes we try to hide in the past. Some of us seek our lost manhood in the arms of another woman.

Andropause from the Inside: One Man's Story

Over the years I have worked with thousands of men going through andropause. Jake's story is unique only in his ability to articulate his feelings more easily than most of us.

Jake is a 45-year-old man. He is married, the father of four grown children. He has been a truck driver for most of his adult life. He came to me because his marriage was in trouble as a result of an affair he had. But as we talked, it became clear that the underlying problems had to do with the changes associated with andropause.

> I think things really started with my depression, though I didn't recognize it at the time. I can now understand what depression really is. Not since I was a child did I feel such a deep-seated anger and sadness. I would yell and I would cry. I couldn't believe it was me. Here I was, a 45-year-old grown man, a truck driver, throwing a tantrum like a 4-year-old or bawling like a baby.
>
> Looking back now I can see that the depression preceded the affair by two years, though at the time I didn't feel depressed. It felt more like everyone else went out of their way to irritate me. I loved my wife, but the passion seemed to be draining out of our relationship. I didn't realize it was really the passion draining out of me.
>
> My thinking began to change. I told myself I wasn't getting enough of what I needed, but I didn't know how to ask for what was important to me. I felt like my manhood was slipping away and I didn't know what to do.

That was when I started noticing the 28-year-old waitress who began to work at one of the restaurants I often stopped at when I was on the road. She was interested in me. She found me attractive. I felt complimented. I felt wanted. At that time my wife and I had just come through some hard times and now had two of our grown children living with us. I think I carried some bitterness toward her and my kids for a situation that I didn't seem to have any control over. It's awful to feel powerless over a situation.

So I had a chance for something that I thought I would never have a chance at again. How many guys pushing 50 would in their wildest dreams have a girl, that young and attractive, come after them?

I took it. I know now that I absolutely should not have. What a high price to pay, to risk the loss of my marriage, for such a short-lived pleasure. But it ended as quickly as it started. And the truth is I honestly did love my wife.

Yet I still felt a deep discontent. The depression came back—light gauge at first, but it got worse as time went on. I started having a hard time with details. I was working on remodeling the attic and couldn't seem to do the job right. I was impatient and wouldn't take the time to read the directions and do the measurements correctly. It just became too much for me. The project still remains, to this day, unfinished.

I seem to have lost my "can-do" attitude. It has been replaced by worry, unsureness, and doubt. I feel I have lost my self-confidence and belief in myself.

That was another thing I found that drew me to the younger woman. She gave me a renewed sense of power, a clear sense of direction. She made me feel strong and important. I felt important. We were important to each other. I felt needed again.

With my spouse I often felt awkward, like two teenagers who don't know how to kiss and bump noses and arms. I felt like we were walking on eggshells, afraid to make the wrong move. I felt like I couldn't do anything right, that as a man I was a complete klutz, if not a failure. I never felt that with the younger woman.

One of the most difficult aspects of this time of life is the uncertainty. I question everything. I have faith in nothing. Even though I hate the way I feel, I can't seem to help it.

To make a long story short, my wife's detective work and my sloppy sneaking around brought my three-month affair to an end.

I can see things in my wife now that I have been blind to for the past 14 years. It's amazing to me that I could close my eyes and

> refuse to see the obvious for so long. In the end, some years from now, whichever way this story goes, I will never doubt that my wife really loved me. She has dealt with her deep heartache without making me feel even worse than I do.
>
> She has tried in every way possible to help me get through this mysterious emotional passage. I know now how devastating my affair was to my wife and to our marriage. When a marriage suffers such a potentially deadly blow, and when the one who took that blow turns her attention to the healing of her attacker, I think it can only be real love at work.

After more than a year in therapy it looks like Jake and his wife are on a positive path. Although there is still a lot of healing that needs to occur before full trust will be restored, the couple is committed to each other and to making the marriage work. They both acknowledge that this is has been the most difficult time of their lives, but feel they are on the way to the life that they both have wanted. Both feel very thankful that they stayed together during these tough times and that Jake could recognize that he was going through andropause.

If you think you are going through andropause, follow the program in this book so you can live long and well.

PART II

The Problem with Men's Health

CHAPTER 4

Why Men Die Sooner and Live Sicker

He is playing by the rules of the male game plan and with lemming-like purpose he is destroying himself—emotionally, psychologically and physically.

—Herb Goldberg

When we got the call from Betsy I was shocked. She told us that her husband, Thomas, had just died of a heart attack. It didn't seem possible. We had visited with them recently and Thomas didn't seem to be a man about to have a heart attack. He had just turned 50 and was in good health. He walked regularly and ate well. That could have been me, I thought. So what happened?

I found out he had died pursuing one of his passions, picking blackberries that Betsy made into her rich and wonderful cobblers which we had shared many times with them. I pictured us all sitting around the table eating cobbler and ice cream. For the first time I saw in my mind Thomas's big belly. He never seemed fat to me, just pleasantly plump. Knowing that a number of his arteries had become clogged made me see his passion for cobbler and his plumpness in a new way.

I also remembered that Thomas had been more withdrawn than I remembered him. Betsy said he was having difficulty accepting the fact that he was getting older and couldn't do some of the physical things that he had once been able to do. She confided that he was questioning his future and what he wanted to do with his life and was concerned that he seemed to be stuck in neutral. She was worried that he might be depressed.

Thomas had always been somewhat reserved. He wasn't the kind of guy to open up and talk about his feelings easily. Like so many men I've known over the years, both personally and professionally, he suffered in silence. His death woke me up and made me aware of the destructive patterns that so many of us experience in our lives from birth until death.

The following points stand out:

- Women around the world have a survival advantage over men—sometimes by as much as 10 years.
- In the United States life expectancy at birth is about 79 years for women and about 72 years for men.
- The death rates for women are lower than those for men at all ages—even before birth. Though 115 males are conceived for every 100 females, males begin an immediate slide and just 104 boys are born for every 100 girls.
- By age 25 women outnumber men, and the trend continues throughout the life span. By the time men and women reach the century mark, for every 100 females there are only 19 males.
- Men are almost seven times as likely as women to report chronic drinking and more than three times as many men report binge drinking.
- Men have a higher death rate for every one of the top 15 leading causes of death.

Men's health expert Dr. Aaron Kipnis offers the following statistics to illustrate the social destructiveness that males experience:

- Seventy percent of all assault victims are male.
- Eighty percent of homicide victims are male.
- Eighty-five percent of the homeless are male.
- Ninety percent of people with AIDS are male.
- Ninety-three percent of people killed on the job are male.
- Ninety-five percent of people in prisons and jails are male.

ACTION OPTION

The statistics tell us about averages, about trends, about what's going on with "men." What do the statistics have to do with you and me? Write down the three statistics that are of greatest concern to you. Pick one that you'd like to learn more about.

Commit to gathering information over the next month and doing something to help improve things for the better.

—⚬⚬—

It should be clear by now that we aren't doing so well taking care of ourselves. But why is that? Throughout the book, we will be exploring that question and what we can do about it. To begin, let's examine our health practices.

Men's Health Practices Are Unhealthy

Until recently most people accepted the fact that men's bodies break down sooner than women's. We believed it was merely a part of our nature. Though some of the difference may result from simply being male, a great deal results from the way we live.

Based on recent research, men's health leader Will Courtenay found 10 key factors that contribute to men's loss of health as they age:

1. We are less likely to practice self-care.

One recent study of a random sample of 6,000 health maintenance organization members found that 77 percent of the women conducted self-screenings for cancer compared to 45 percent of the men.

Sleep is another form of self-care, and we get far less sleep than women do. Even among a national sample of 11,000 health-conscious respondents, the men reported sleeping an average of 6 hours to women's 8.21. The fact that we sleep fewer hours than women contributes to our significantly higher injury rates. Each year, sleepiness is believed to cause 17,000 nighttime injury deaths, 3,500 unintentional injury deaths, and over half of all work-related injury deaths.

Additionally, there is growing evidence that immune function decreases with even modest sleep deprivation. Our poorer quality of sleep also increases our health risks. For example, sleep apnea, which is often associated with snoring, increases the risk of heart attack 23 times in men.

2. Our diets are worse than women's.

Males consume more saturated fat and dietary cholesterol than females do, even when sex differences are adjusted for body size. We are less likely than women to limit fat or red meat in our diets.

We eat far fewer fruits and vegetables than women and consume less fiber. We more often skip breakfast and are less likely to limit sugar and sweet foods in our diets. We also drink far more coffee than women and are more likely to drink at least five cups each day.

Poor diet, along with a sedentary lifestyle, accounts for an estimated 300,000 deaths each year. The "Male American Diet" is a major contributor to heart disease and cancer, the leading killers of men in the United States.

3. More men than women are overweight.

Contrary to popular belief, men have more problems with weight than women. The Department of Health and Human Services defines being significantly overweight as weighing at least 20 percent above ideal body weight. One-third of adults nationally are, by this definition, overweight, and the majority of these are men.

Furthermore, only half as many men as women, at most, attempt to lose weight. Maintaining desirable weight is unequivocally associated with better health and lower mortality rates. In one recent study, men with waists of at least 40 inches were nearly three times as likely to develop heart disease as men with 34-inch waists.

4. We are less physically active than women.

Among those aged 35 to 54, far more men than women engage in little or no physical activity. Among those who are active, women are more likely to engage in light to moderate exercise, which experts agree and research shows is optimal for the body's well-being.

Those of us who *are* active are more likely to be "weekend warriors" who engage in infrequent but strenuous physical activity such as jogging, playing tennis, shoveling snow, or mowing the lawn. In one recent study, those of us who engaged in these strenuous but infrequent activities increased our risk of heart attack 100 times.

There is overwhelming and consistent evidence that *moderate* physical activity significantly reduces the risk of major chronic diseases and premature death. Twelve percent of all deaths are attributable to lack of regular physical activity.

Those of us who are inactive are two to three times more likely to die from any cause than our more active peers. Over one-third of all heart disease deaths are attributed to physical inactivity, more than those attributed to smoking, excess weight, or hypertension.

5. We drink more and use more drugs.

The use of alcohol and other drugs is far greater among men than women. For example, over twice as many of us have used cocaine and five times more men than women drink an average of two or more alcoholic drinks per day. Research consistently reveals greater problem and heavy drinking among men and a higher prevalence of alcohol abuse and dependence.

Tobacco use accounts for roughly one in five deaths overall, and one in four deaths among those aged 35 to 64 years. Twice as many male as female deaths are attributed to smoking, and our higher lifetime use of tobacco is considered a primary reason for our higher rates of cardiovascular disease and stroke.

Each year, nearly one-half million people die of cancer due to tobacco use, and the majority of them are men. Three out of four of us who get any kind of cancer are smokers.

6. We engage in more risk-taking than do women.

Men are more likely than women to drive dangerously. Motor vehicle–related fatalities account for nearly half of all unintentional injury deaths, and men are 2.5 times more likely to die in accidents than are women.

We are far more likely than women to participate in risky sports and recreational activities. It has been suggested that sports injuries pose a greater public health risk than many reportable infectious diseases. It is estimated that 3 to 5 million sports injuries are sustained annually in the United States, the great majority to males.

We begin sexual activity earlier than women and are more likely to engage in high-risk sex. Each day, 33,000 Americans become infected with STDs (sexually transmitted diseases), and sexual behavior accounted for an estimated 30,000 deaths in 1990. Based on a variety of behaviors, including condom use and number of sexual partners, we are much more likely than women to be in the highest risk group for AIDS and other STDs.

7. We engage in more violence.

Our willingness to engage in overt physical aggression contributes to our health risks. We are much more likely than women to be both the perpetrators and the victims of violence.

For example, nearly half of men nationally have been punched or beaten by another person, compared to one-quarter of women.

Fighting is the most immediate antecedent behavior for a great proportion of homicides. The homicide death rate is four times greater for men than women.

Firearm-related injuries are seven times greater among males than females. Nearly 40,000 deaths a year are due to firearms. Ninety per-rent of these are male, including the 9 of 10 deaths that are considered accidents.

8. We have fewer social supports than women.

We have fewer, less intimate friendships than women and are less likely to have a close confidant, particularly someone other than a spouse. Some researchers have even concluded that most of us have no close friends at all.

There is consistent evidence that the lack of social relationships constitutes a risk factor for mortality—especially for us guys. Those of us with the lowest levels of social relationships are two to three times more likely to die from all causes.

In one study of heart disease patients, 50 percent of those without a confidant were dead after five years compared to only 17 percent of those with a spouse or confidant. Those of us with higher levels of social support also maintain more positive health practices. We are likelier to modify unhealthy behavior and adhere to medical treatment. Our immune systems function better and react to stress more efficiently.

9. We have higher risks on the job than women and suffer more when we lose our jobs.

Most jobs in America are demarcated by sex. The vast majority of secretaries, receptionists, child-care professionals, nurses, and salespeople, for instance, are women. Work in timber cutting, fishing, mining, construction, truck driving, farming, and forestry is done almost exclusively by men. Ninety-five percent of all local and state police officers are male, as are the vast majority of firefighters.

Many women are clamoring to break down the sex barriers to employment in traditionally male professions in the hopes of getting better pay and more interesting and varied work experiences. Most are not aware of the higher risks in these "male" professions.

While we constitute 56 percent of the workforce, we account for 94 percent of all fatal injuries on the job. The five industries with the greatest percentage of workers exposed to hazardous chemicals, for instance, are construction, agriculture, oil and gas extraction, and water transportation—all with jobs held primarily by men.

Unemployment is consistently linked with a variety of negative health effects, and there is evidence that these negative effects are greater for men than women. Suicide rates, for instance, are linked with unemployment and economic depression for men, but not for women.

10. We visit physicians less and have far fewer health checkups than women do.

Regular health care visits and screenings were found to be important contributors to our health and longevity, yet according to Kenneth Goldberg, M.D., we make 150 million fewer doctor visits a year than women. Regular screenings, for instance, can detect a variety of cancers at an early stage, when successful treatment is more likely. Ninety percent of cancers that are found when they are still localized are curable.

Even when we manage to get to the doctor, we don't do a very good job in getting the most out of the visit. Most of us lie to our doctors.

- Over 25 percent of us lie because we tell ourselves it is easier than telling the truth.
- Another 25 percent of us lie because we are afraid the doctor will get mad.
- Almost 35 percent of us lie because we are too embarrassed.
- Twenty percent of us lie because we do not want bad news.

We don't just lie about little things, either. Our lies cover topics ranging from following the doctor's advice and taking medications properly to sexual practices and symptoms of a major illness.

Can you imagine a guy who rarely took his car in for a routine checkup, lied to his mechanic about what the problem was, and refused to follow the mechanic's advice on how best to keep the car running well?

When we start taking care of our health at least as well as we take care of our cars, we will go a long way to living more joyous and healthy lives.

ACTION OPTION

Eliminate a Health Risk Now

Go over the 10 factors listed above. Pick one that you are ready to act upon. Do something this week that is supportive of your health. For instance, you may decide to get a health checkup, change your eating habits, or get more exercise. Take an action and see how you feel. You'll be glad you did.

CHAPTER 5

The 14 Emotional and Biological Reasons Men Don't Take Better Care of Themselves

> It was a great mistake, my being born a man. I would have been much more successful as a sea gull or a fish. As it is, I will always be a stranger who never feels at home, who does not really want and is not really wanted, who can never belong, who must always be a little in love with death.
>
> —Eugene O'Neill, *Long Day's Journey into Night*

After working with thousands of men over the last 35 years, I've identified the major reasons that prevent us from living long and well. Some of these will seem obvious once I point them out to you. Others are subtler and will require us to look more deeply to understand how they affect us. I believe that the truth will set us free and allow us to live fuller and more joyful lives.

1. We don't know the facts of life.

Many studies have shown that we are less interested in health issues than women. If we're less interested in a subject we will be less likely to keep up on the latest information about it. Most of us are more interested in the health of our automobiles than the health of our bodies.

As a result, we know more about the function and workings of carburetors than we know about the function and workings of our prostates. We understand that when the little red light goes on in the car, it means "danger." We know something is wrong and know where to look to fix it. Yet we can have back pains, chest pains, blood in our urine, or other "red light" signals and ignore them.

Most of us would never see the red danger signal in our cars, hit our hand against the dash until the light went out, then drive merrily along believing we had solved the problem. Yet we will routinely drink or take drugs, take antacids or aspirin, to cover our pain and assume that everything is OK with our health because we no longer notice the warning signal that is meant to inform us that something is wrong.

We understand that our car needs regular checkups and usually check the oil, water, fan belts, and so on periodically so that we know if something needs to be added or fixed. Yet we will avoid, like the plague, regular health checkups to test PSA for prostate problems or our blood pressure to alert us to possible heart problems.

"He runs his body while it's the equivalent of three quarts low," says Ken Goldberg, M.D., director of the Male Health Center, talking about most of us men. "One reason men don't think about routine maintenance for their bodies is that they know next to nothing about what makes them work."

2. Taking Care of Ourselves Is Seen As Unmanly.

From the time we are little we are taught that "boys don't cry," that asking for help is a sign of weakness and that injury is a badge of courage.

I still remember the early warnings from my father and sometimes from my mother. As a rough-and-tumble three-year-old I was always getting a skinned elbow or knee and would howl to high heaven when I got hurt. But I was told, sometimes gently, other times harshly, that "big boys don't cry." I learned that to be male was to be strong. I found I got praise when I suffered in silence and rejection when I cried out too loudly or too often.

When I was in my early teens we played football after school and on weekends. I was the smallest kid on the team and felt I had to act tough in order to be accepted. I would tackle boys twice my weight and prided myself on my ability to shake the opposition. One day, playing at a nearby school where we had to scale a large fence to get inside, I ran for a touchdown carrying three bigger boys on my back. When I was finally tackled I felt a sharp pain in my left shoulder as the weight of the boys crushed me into the turf.

When I got up I had grass in my mouth, cuts on my face, an arm that didn't hang right, and the praise of all the guys on both teams. I quickly wiped the blood off my face, gave my arm a couple of practice stretches, and returned to the game. It wasn't until everyone had decided to quit for the day that I was forced to admit that I was injured. I simply couldn't lift my weight to climb over the fence. With guys razzing me that I was a "wimp," three of the larger boys pushed me up the fence and helped me to drop over the other side.

When I got home, my mother saw the pain on my face and asked what was wrong. "Nothing," I replied. "Just a few bruises from playing ball." I took a shower and tried to ignore the pain, which was now excruciating, the swelling that was making my arm look like a sack of potatoes, and the awful blue-black color that spread out from my shoulder and traveled down my arm.

The next day was Sunday, and I couldn't get out of bed. My mother kept asking what was wrong, and I kept evading her questions. Finally, she insisted on seeing the arm. "Get up, get dressed. I'm taking you to the emergency room," she said in no uncertain terms. I was somewhat irritated. I was sure I was OK and didn't need any doctor to tell me I just needed to rest. I was also relieved that someone was taking charge of getting me help.

The doctor in the emergency room took a quick look and asked me to move my arm. I made a manly gesture of raising it over my head and nearly fainted. He ordered Xrays and found that I had badly dislocated my shoulder. He manipulated the shoulder back into place while I nearly ground my teeth down trying not to scream or cry. He said I might need surgery later, but they'd have to wait and see how it healed. I wore a sling to school for the next six weeks and was the envy of all the guys for my battlefield bravery. The damaged shoulder was my medal. It was admired by both the boys and girls.

—ꝏ—

It isn't until we move into middle age that we begin to question these beliefs, usually as a result of recognizing the debilitation that those early injuries cause as we get older.

Since it wasn't often clear exactly what it meant to be manly, we learned that an easy way to feel like a man was do the opposite of what the females did. If the girls were soft and gentle, the boys were tough and aggressive. If the girls talked quietly, the boys played noisy games. If the girls read magazines on self-care, the boys, of course, could not. We had to read war stories and adventure novels.

3. We Learn to Deny and Ignore All Pain.

From the time we are boys we are taught to pretend that we are not hurt, even though we may be in terrible pain. When we are hurt playing ball we are taught to shake it off and get back in the game. The high school hero at our school was the boy who played the second half of the basketball game on a broken ankle. He never complained.

"Men," says Royda Crose, author of *Why Women Live Longer Than Men,* "are more at risk of early death because they are taught to ignore weakness, illness, and health concerns. . . . They not only don't listen to their bodies, but they are applauded for the denial of pain and discomfort."

Trained to ignore pain and play hurt, we develop the belief that the best way to stay healthy is to ignore any signs of ill health. Even to practice prevention is to acknowledge that there are problems we want to prevent from occurring. We're like children with the magical belief that if we look at something scary we will make it real and dangerous. If we refuse to look at it, it will magically disappear.

We need to learn that this kind of magic is destructive and counterproductive. In fact, ignoring signs of trouble can be dangerous. Preventing problems before they occur can save our lives.

4. Illness Equals Weakness Equals Unmanliness.

If we ignore pain, it is easy to believe that our bodies are invincible. We identify with our action figures that are perfect and strong all the time. In our younger days, we seemed to be invincible. Injuries healed overnight even after we had given ourselves a beating. Colds and the flu usually went away by themselves, as if by magic. It never occurred to us that it was because our bodies were young and healthy and needed care to stay that way. We just thought that being a man meant being strong and having a body that lasted forever.

For many of us getting sick or hurt is a sign of weakness. It's as though catching a cold or the flu is an indication that we aren't trying hard enough, that we are losing the battle with the germs that are attacking us. In our upbringing, being strong was a mark of manhood. Being weak was for sissies, those who were less than men. As we get older and we begin to lose our physical stamina and strength there is a great fear that we are losing our manhood. If illness may set us on the slippery slide to losing our manliness, we best ignore any signs of illness.

5. We're Afraid of Giving Up Control.

No one likes to feel that he or she is out of control. But men have a particularly difficult time. Women learn early on that there are things about their bodies that are beyond their control. They have a monthly period, whether they like it or not. There are clear physical and emotional changes that "just happen."

We also have hormonal cycles and emotional changes throughout the month, even though we don't have a menstrual cycle. But we deny such changes. We do everything we can to control events in our lives and even try and control our body functions. Attempting to control parts of ourselves that are beyond control, we build up fear.

Acknowledging an illness—even going to a doctor—forces us to let our guard down, to become vulnerable to another human being. Many of us would rather die than let ourselves be vulnerable. What often kills us is our inability to give up control and allow others to help us.

6. We Are Secretly Proud of Our Wounds.

Even as boys, our cuts and scratches were seen by other boys and girls as badges of courage. Although we ignored the pain and suffering that went with them, we got a sense of pride in displaying our wounds. I remember when I hurt my leg playing basketball and was placed in a hip-length cast for two months. My status in my group of peers went up a few notches. I got sympathy from the girls and admiration from the guys.

A few years ago, I attended a men's conference with 300 other men. In one of the exercises we were given strips of red cloth and were asked to tie them in places on our bodies where we had been hurt or wounded. The room quickly turned red. Each man had multiple ties on all parts of his body. As we talked and the tears of frustration and sadness were released, it became apparent that what were once badges of courage and honor in our youth had become marks of pain and shame as we had gotten older.

No one was cheering us as we touched scars from football injuries and operations. We wished we had taken better care of ourselves in our youth. Many of us had to live with irreparable damage. We all vowed to do a better job taking care of ourselves in the future.

7. Parental Training Encourages Us to Suppress Our Emotions.

Most parents believe they treat their infant sons and daughters the same. The truth is, they don't. Studies show that infant boys are touched and cuddled less than infant girls. Physical contact with boys usually involves stimulation. There are bounces, tickles, and rough play. With girls there is more gentle contact and soft words.

As early as their sons' first year, mothers tend to spend less time with their little boys. By the time they are a year and a half boys are left to play alone more often and for longer periods of time than little girls.

We learn early that emotions are not for us. Parents talk in more action-oriented language to their sons, in more emotion-oriented language to daughters. When emotions are discussed with boys, it is usually about anger rather than hurt or fear.

So we learn early on to disconnect from our feelings, except perhaps from our anger. It doesn't take long before our feelings are buried so deep they become unavailable to us. In later years when we're asked, "How do you feel?" we don't have a clue. And since feelings are the key elements in our body's early warning system, letting us know when something is wrong—or when something is right, for that matter—we often don't know when something is going wrong until very late in the game.

8. Kids in the Neighborhood Enforce Unhealthy Gender Roles.

Once boys and girls are in school, traditional gender roles are enforced by peers even more strictly than by adults. Girls who don't tow the line are ignored while boys are ridiculed and attacked physically. Being accused of being a "tomboy" carries much less vehemence than being accused of being a "sissy."

I remember coming to school one day when I was eight or nine wearing a pair of jeans that had a little bit of elastic in the back. I liked them, and they were quite comfortable. I wasn't in school an hour before my new jeans were discovered by some of the boys who teased me mercilessly, insisting that I was wearing girls' jeans. In those early years, to do anything that might mark you as a "sissy" or "acting like a girl" was to be teased into oblivion. Most of us learned the lessons well.

9. Experiences in the Locker Room Teach Us to Feel Bad About Our Bodies.

For many young men the locker room is a place of terror. We are never more vulnerable than when we have to take our clothes off and let it all hang out. If our body is different in any way, we can be the brunt of vicious teasing. If we are gay, suspected of being gay, or act in any way that might seem effeminate we are subject to being physically abused.

I remember being teased mercilessly as a young adolescent because I began to get hair on my body earlier than most of my peers. Some guy would invariably sneak up on me and grab a pinch of my genital hair and laugh and taunt me. The other boys would join in the "fun." Not only was it physically painful, but emotionally humiliating. Later, as the other boys matured physically, I was teased because I was shorter than most of them.

I learned to hate my body and wished I could just look like everyone else. It laid the foundation for my later life willingness to "punish" my body, though it took me years to recognize the connection between my early shame and my later self-destructive behavior.

We all learned the lesson. Don't complain, play hurt, ignore the pain, forget your future, win now. Many of us carry those destructive lessons throughout our lives.

10. Males in the Media Teach Us to be "Strong and Silent."

The movies and television depict the ultimate male superhero as a man who puts himself in harm's way, takes inordinate risks to protect beautiful women, and is immune to being hurt. When I was growing up our male media models were the cowboys—Tom Mix, Gene Autry, John Wayne. They were strong and silent, kept their feelings to themselves, and solved problems with a gun. One of my favorites of the time was the Lone Ranger. In addition to the values of power, silence, and violence, he taught us that real men hid behind a mask and were loners. If there was anyone we might trust, it was a subordinate male who did our bidding without question.

Not a whole lot has changed for those growing up today. Now the superheroes are "Make My Day" Clint Eastwood, "Indiana Jones" Harrison Ford, "Rocky" Sylvester Stallone, and "Jimmy the Tulip" Bruce Willis. They are not quite as silent, but much more violent. They still court danger, but never really get hurt. Few even have a sidekick to keep them company, and so they make the Lone Ranger look like a social butterfly. These are not exactly great role models for promoting men's health. We frequently hear about women being relegated to lower-paying jobs like secretary and receptionist and their desire to break through the "male-only" barrier to claim jobs that are more interesting and higher paying. But we usually fail to recognize that most of these "male only" jobs are not really all that great.

11. Guys at Work Learn to Die Like Real Men.

When *The Jobs Rated Almanac* ranked 250 jobs from best to worst based on a combination of salary, stress, work environment, outlook, security, safety, and physical demands, they found that 24 of the 25 worst jobs were almost all male jobs.

These included such jobs as truck driver, sheet-metal worker, roofer, boilermaker, lumberjack, construction worker, machinery operator, welder, and ironworker. All of these "worst jobs" have one thing in common: they are detrimental to health, and they are performed by men 95 to 100 percent of the time.

Every day, almost as many men are killed at work as were killed on the average day during the Vietnam War. Every workday *hour,* one construction worker in the United States loses his life. The more hazardous the job, the greater the percentage of men. For instance, fire fighting is 99 percent male, logging is 98 percent male, heavy trucking is 98 percent male, construction is 98 percent male, and coal mining is 97 percent male. It's not surprising that Warren Farrell, author of *The Myth of Male Power,* calls men's work "The Death Professions."

It doesn't take much awareness to recognize that most garbage collectors are men. But most people are probably not aware that a garbageman is two and a half times more likely to be killed than a police officer and that 70 percent of the collection crew in an average city sustained job-related injuries in the last year alone.

Most men take these jobs not because they are desirable, but because they feel they need to take them in order to support their wives and children.

But men don't just die from "dangerous jobs"; they also die from the stress caused by overwork at regular "safe" jobs. The Japanese call it *karoshi*—death from overwork. In the past 20 years in Japan, sudden deaths among top executives have increased 1,400 percent. A survey by the Japanese government found that executives *average* 70 hours per week. With the expansion of world markets and the need to be competitive, top executives in countries all over the world literally kill themselves to remain on top.

One way to look at the perks given to mostly male chief executives is to see them as bribes to sacrifice their individuality, their health, and even their life in the service of business success.

12. Females Help Reinforce Our Tough Guy Image.

I still remember a cartoon I saw as a young man. It was in *Playboy* magazine and showed a good-looking young woman sitting across from a solid, stoic-looking man. The woman had just taken a fork and stuck it into the bridge of the man's nose. He sits there without comment and without any show of pain. The caption reads, "That's what I love about you, Louie, you're tough."

In our youthful antiwar years protesting the killing in Vietnam, there was a slogan we heard: "Women say 'yes' to men who say 'no.'" It was the hope of all us male marchers that opposing the war would make us seem sexy to women. It may have worked for war resister David Harris, who attracted and later married Joan Baez, but the reality for most of us was that women were still more attracted to the roughneck than to the peacenik.

I remember that in junior high and high school, the best-looking and most-desirable girls always went out with the "hoods" or the "jocks." They even went out with the guys who treated them badly. I couldn't understand it. I was nice, courteous, and thoughtful. I treated girls with respect and care. I had lots of girl friends, but few girlfriends. I learned that girls liked guys who were tough and aggressive.

The most popular guys were the football players who "kicked ass" each weekend and were found with their arms around the waists of the prettiest girls during the week. It was clear that if you wanted to get the most desirable girls, it was best to knock heads on the sports field or be willing to bash a head or get your own head bashed in after-school fights.

13. Mating Strategies Make Men Risk Their Health.

From a genetic perspective, it is less important whether we survive to a ripe old age than whether we reproduce. Less well known than Darwin's ideas on how natural selection works to produce species differences were his ideas on reproduction and what he called "sexual selection."

The idea that reproduction was the key to understanding why we do what we do was ignored for many years after Darwin's death and has only recently come back into vogue. "Its principal insight," says Matt Ridley, author of *The Red Queen: Sex and the Evolution of Human Nature,* "is that the goal of an animal is not just to survive but to breed. Indeed, where breeding and survival come into conflict, it is breeding that takes precedence; for example, salmon starve to death while breeding. And breeding, in sexual species, consists of finding an appropriate partner and persuading it to part with a package of genes."

From an evolutionary perspective, if endangering our health enabled us to be more reproductively successful, these traits would be passed down through succeeding generations. To understand how this occurs we need to take a look at what it means to be male and what it means to be female.

Throughout our ancestral past, in order to get close to a female, a male must first complete with other males. Whether the male is a lion, a bull elephant, a hummingbird, or a human, he will tend toward greater aggression so that he can best his competition. It isn't surprising that men are most aggressive and competitive with other males when they are between the ages of 14 and 28, the prime reproductive years.

Once a male has gotten access to a female he must convince her that he is worthy of her attention. Throughout the world and across cultures women are drawn to men who have resources.

A man will take jobs that are dangerous, put in long hours of overtime, even work himself to death in order to find and keep a woman. He won't often be conscious of this fact. For him, he overworks because that's what a man does. But his evolutionary history plays a role.

Humans inherit many things from our ancestors—the color of our eyes, our height, whether we lose our hair, and how to eat, think, and speak. But above all we inherit a drive to reproduce. Therefore, anything that increased the chances of a person reproducing successfully was passed on at the expense of anything else. "We can confidently assert," says Matt Ridley, "that there is nothing in our natures that was not carefully 'chosen' in this way for its ability to contribute to eventual reproductive success."

Bottom line: We will often do whatever it takes to get and keep a woman. If it means endangering our health, we will do it. Remember, none of our direct ancestors died childless. Think for a moment of the power contained in that statement. Over the period of a billion years of sexual selection, not one of our ancestors dropped the ball.

Men are often scolded when we don't take better care of ourselves. The underlying message seems to be "What's the matter with you that you can't do a simple thing like remembering to take your vitamins, or driving more slowly, or eating more fruits and vegetables." Believe me, men aren't dumb. We will always act in what we perceive as our best interests. I have found that the most critical reason we don't take better care of ourselves is the shame that we experience throughout our lives.

14. Shame: The Main Barrier to Men's Health.

Over the years of working with men I found it very helpful to become aware of the self-destructive behavior that is so much a part of men's lives. When I worked with men in therapy it was also useful for me to help them understand the underlying beliefs that contributed to their unhealthy lifestyles.

However, there seemed to be another level that I wasn't touching. I understood that beliefs such as "Taking care of myself is unmanly," "I must be willing to die like a man," and "I must keep my true feelings buried inside" contributed to our unhealthy practices. But I couldn't help wondering what the underlying cause of these beliefs was. I realized eventually that the cause was shame, and that is the subject of the next chapter.

CHAPTER 6

Men's Shame

Shame is feeling alone in the pit of unworthiness.

—Merle Fossum

WE LIVE IN A shame-based culture where more and more of us feel a loss of respect. Many of us sell our souls to get or hold a job. Others have no hope of ever finding work that can give our lives meaning.

As we move into the second half of life many of us feel disheartened about the changes that we experience in our bodies, minds, and souls. We often feel like we're over the hill and useless. Instead of being proud mentors and guides to younger men, we hang our heads in shame. Yet more and more young men are starving for the care and respect that only their elders can give them.

Many young men would kill to get respect or to keep from losing the little they have. Many do. "The prison inmates I work with have told me repeatedly, when I asked them why they had assaulted someone," says James Gilligan, M.D., an expert on male shame and violence, "that it was because 'he disrespected me. . . .' The word 'disrespect' is so central in the vocabulary, moral value system, and psychodynamics of these chronically violent men that they have abbreviated it into the slang term, 'he dissed me.'"

The hunger for respect is something that is so apparent with men in prison that we have come to accept, if not totally understand, it. Yet this is a hunger that many of us experience every day. Most of us discount our feelings of being "dissed." We assume that we are too strong, that our skin is too thick, that the slights are too minor. Yet we can't hide the fact that we are deeply affected.

One of things many women and men are most confused about is that things will be going along well, when out of the blue a man will react with anger. Or a couple will be in a long-term relationship and all of a sudden he decides he has to get out. Over the years I have come to see that these sudden outbursts, or changes in direction, are often the result of accumulated shame.

During the 32 years I worked with clients having drug abuse problems, I found that the core experience driving their hunger for drugs was shame. Most all felt there was a deep wound, a "black hole," at the center of their being. Shame was the feeling associated with this loss. "There is a hole at my core," said one addict, "where my self ought to be." Drugs were often used in a futile attempt to fill the void.

We see the same dynamic with violence. "The emotion of shame is the primary or ultimate cause of all violence," says Gilligan, "whether toward others or toward the self." Our unwillingness to take better care of ourselves is a form of self-destructiveness. It is violence turned inward and is related to shame.

For most of us, shame is deeply hidden, and the things that trigger shame often seem insignificant. For many, shame is set off by experiences that seem so minor few people would believe a person is affected. A funny look, a tone of voice, or a forgotten item from the grocery store can set us off.

The shame that many of us will do anything to hide is how easily we are shamed. "This is a secret that many of them would rather die than reveal," says Gilligan. "The secret is that they feel ashamed—deeply ashamed, chronically ashamed, acutely ashamed, over matters that are so trivial that their very triviality makes it even more shameful to feel ashamed about them."

Many of us grew up in families and communities that put us down and undermined our self-respect so often and so consistently that it takes almost nothing to push us over the edge. We hunger for a kind word—to be told that we are smart, or good, or needed, or appreciated. Often, we are like beggars. We are deeply ashamed, both of our neediness and the ease with which our hunger can be triggered.

What Is This Shame That Men Share?

"Shame," says author Merle Fossum, "is feeling alone in the pit of unworthiness." He describes shame as being much more deeply rooted than most people believe. "Shame is not just a low reading on the thermometer of self-esteem," he says. "Shame is something like cancer—it grows on its own momentum." Both shame and guilt are ways people experience feeling bad. Yet the two are quite different. Guilt involves feeling bad about what we do or fail to do. Shame is feeling bad about who we are, about our very being. The shame that men experience is a kind of soul murder, undermining the foundations of our masculine selves.

Until we are willing to confront the sources of our shame we will always have difficulty taking good care of ourselves. If we feel unworthy at the core of our being, we will always find ways to undermine our health. Shame is such a distasteful emotion that we tend to deny we even feel it.

The Roots of Men's Shame

Shame is such a difficult and fearful emotion that most of us erase it from our consciousness as soon as it emerges. However, rather than going away, it becomes buried deeper and deeper in our consciousness. It is like a wound that doesn't heal, but simply gets covered over. Although we may look fine, and the skin over the wound may heal, inside there is an infection that continually poisons our system and sense of well-being.

The nature of shame is such that many of us would literally rather die than reveal the sources of our pain. It's why so many of us suffer in silence and why we find it so difficult to take good care of ourselves despite our resolutions. Shame acts like a silent thief stealing our resolve and our hope for a better future. To get to our true self that is the source of our health-giving nature, we have to be willing to let go of our "look-good" image and confront the sources of our shame.

I have found that there are six primary sources of our shame. See which ones you identify with. But remember it is easy to deny our shame. It takes a great deal of courage to move into and through our shame.

The Shame of Being Seen as Less Valuable than Females

I was sitting in front of the TV watching one of the old classic black-and-white movies. There was the scene where the ocean liner is sinking. The lifeboats are being lowered and everyone is moving toward the boats, trying to keep their panic under control. The traditional shout rings out: "Women and children first."

This scene is such an accepted part of our experience that few of us stop to ask why women's lives are more valuable than men's.

Though we feel pride at being the protectors of women and children, I believe we feel a deep sense of shame that our lives are expendable.

The Shame of Violence and Addiction

We generally think of civilization as being a very good thing, a wonderful achievement of human beings that elevated us above our barbarous past. Though there are many benefits we have derived since the dawn of the Agricultural Revolution in 8000 B.C., there have also been many drawbacks.

We have experienced huge population increases, the eradication of tribal peoples throughout the world, the devastation of the environment, and continuous warfare. We know that the birth of civilization also brought us alcohol and drug abuse.

It is often said that if you want to get a glimpse of people's true priorities, not just what they profess, take a look at how they spend their money. I've often wondered how much the world spends on addiction and death. Carl Sagan has given us an answer. "Every year," he said, "the world spends one trillion dollars on armaments. In addition, the world spends on illegal narcotic drugs something like half a trillion dollars every year. That is capital otherwise unavailable to the human species. We have decided to spend it on war and drugs."

If to the half trillion dollars we spend on "illegal narcotic" drugs we added the money we spend on alcohol, nicotine, gambling, pornography, and other forms of addictive escape, I'm sure the price tag for all our addictions would equal the trillion dollars we spend on war each year.

Although we can point to a great many valuable things civilization has brought us, we must be willing to open our eyes and recognize that the primary, even though unintended, legacy of civilization has been violence and addiction. An unbiased observer of our "civilized" move to agriculture and domestication might conclude, as did Jared Diamond, the Pulitzer Prize–winning author, that it was "the worst mistake in the history of the human race."

The Shame of Our Lost Connection to the Wilderness

As we moved from a hunter-gatherer way of life to one based on domestication of plants and animals, we destroyed much of the wilderness.

Instead of looking at the wilderness in all its sacred beauty, with the dawn of civilization we began to distill, dismiss, discard, and destroy the wilderness. We became interested only in those things that we could use. The rest we threw away. As the ones most connected to the wilderness, it was men who lost the most when the land and the animals became domesticated. Something in our spirit, I believe, dies when the wilderness dies. We experience a deep, primal wound to our souls.

The Shame of Losing Our Roles in Life

For all of human history (as well as our mammalian history) males and females had different primary jobs in bringing into being, and raising, the next generation. Sigmund Freud suggested that women had "penis envy" because they lacked the wondrous organ that only men possess. Given the woman's greater contribution to the emergence and nurturing of life, this belief seems to be more about men's fear of accepting his own envious feelings. It is more likely that men possess a strong "womb and breast envy." We all came from a woman's womb and we all suckled at the breast (at least until our "civilized" practice of offering bottles with rubber nipples instead).

Our contribution to the next generation is as vital as women's, but it is different. If we don't contribute our sperm, there is no chance of pregnancy. Though it may be a tiny sperm we contribute, he's an important little guy, nonetheless. However, where we made our most important contributions was in hunting, protecting, and mentoring. With the advent of our civilized way of life, these traditional male roles began to diminish drastically.

The Loss of Our Role as Hunters During the 4-million-year history of our human journey, it was generally the men who left the safety of the camp and went out into the wild to hunt. These excursions were not just about getting food. In fact, it was the women who gathered most of what was necessary for survival.

The hunt was essentially a spiritual experience. It was a way for men to bond deeply with each other (a bond that has only been approached in modern warfare), to relate to large animals as worthy adversaries, and to put their lives on the line in the service of the tribe.

The loss of the hunt is a hidden shame that often manifests itself in our contemporary culture of violence—violence toward ourselves, other men, women, and the environment. Without the spiritual aspects of the hunt, killing becomes an addiction that continues to feed on itself without end.

The Loss of Our Role as Protectors Being the ones who were physically stronger, we were the ones who took on the primary role of protecting the tribe. Although women could be fierce protectors of their children, they were not as easily suited to protect the group as a whole.

There were four potential points of danger to the tribe: animals, other men, nature, and the supernatural. Just as men hunted large animals, there were some large animals that hunted humans. Women and children who might wander from the safety of the camp were particularly vulnerable. It was the men's job to protect their women and children from becoming food for a hungry lion or tiger.

Since it was the men who ventured into the wilderness, they were the ones who were attuned to changes in the environment that might affect the safety of the tribe. Coming storms, changes in the migration habits of the animals, forest fires, and the like were often noticed first by the men.

Nature and spirit were not seen as separate by our ancestors. Tuning into nature was also a way to connect with the supernatural. Animals were often seen as messengers from the gods. Men, with their particular affinity for animals, were able to intercede on behalf of the tribe to protect all from natural and supernatural dangers.

With the advent of agriculture men's role as protector was lost. The animals became domesticated, and the only wild ones left were in zoos and circuses. Protecting our family from attack by other men turned into wars fought for land, wealth, or abstract principles. Rather than protecting women and children, wars usually caused more pain for them.

When we stopped being partners with nature, but tried to become masters of nature, we lost our protective advantage. We increasingly moved to a state where our attempts to control more and more of the natural world are killing off the very life supports we need to ensure the survival of our families and our communities.

Cut off from nature, we are also cut off from the spiritual world. Our collective loss of faith feeds our shame.

The Loss of Our Role as Mentors One of the most significant and vital functions that men had in hunter-gatherer societies was in mentoring the young, particularly the young men. In fact, most of these cultures believe that a boy cannot become a man without the active intervention of older men.

In the first cross-cultural study of manhood, anthropologist David Gilmore found that becoming a man is a process that requires that a boy undergo an initiation conducted by the men in the tribe. In cultures as diverse as those of Japan, India, China, the Mediterranean lands, aboriginal South America, Oceania, East Africa, ancient Greece, and North America, he found the patterns were similar.

Wherever he studied what it takes to be a man he found that "real manhood is different from simple anatomical maleness . . . that it is not a natural condition that comes about spontaneously through biological maturation but rather is a precarious or artificial state that boys must win against powerful odds." A girl's transition to womanhood is marked by her first menses. A boy has no similar biological marker. He must be initiated by other men.

For boys, the rites of passage were intimately tied in with the hunt. Through the initiation from boyhood to manhood, we learned to put our lives on the line in the service of our people. It was through the hunt—the preparation, tracking the animals, killing, bringing the meat to the tribe, and telling stories—that boys learned the values of manhood. We learned about life and death, courage in the face of danger, dealing with fear, channeling the blood lust of testosterone-induced desire, teamwork, accepting failure, being humble, the exaltation of success, the guilt of killing a fellow being, the recognition that all life is precious, and the knowledge that someday it will be our turn to give our life so that some other creature in nature will live.

With the advent of agriculture we lost many of the vital roles that made us feel like men. Many men I've seen describe this feeling of unmanliness. I've often heard these sentiments: "No matter what I do in the world, no matter how successful I am, no matter how many women I've been to bed with, no matter how expensive a car I drive, in my heart of hearts I don't feel like a man."

When we feel this way, it is very hard to feel that we have something to pass on to younger men. We may see the need to be a mentor, but we don't feel we have the heart for it. Young men feel the loss and grow up without the guidance of older men.

The Shame of Lost Fatherhood The most basic form of male mentoring that we do is being a good father to our children. This function, like many others, has deteriorated over the last 10,000 years of civilization. David Blankenhorn, author of *Fatherless America: Confronting Our Most Urgent Social Problem,* describes our present situation this way: "The United States is becoming an increasingly fatherless society. A generation ago, an American child could reasonably expect to grow up with his or her father. Today, an American child can reasonably expect not to."

In the present dialogue there is a great deal of blame. Many absent fathers blame the women for not allowing them to see their children on a regular basis. Many women blame the fathers for not being more responsible. Some blame the court system for favoring mothers over fathers in custody disputes. Some blame the youth for their lack of respect for their elders. Children are often caught in the middle and suffer greatly, often for the rest of their lives, when parents separate and can't work out healthy ways to parent their children.

Although there is ample evidence to the contrary, many have come to believe that every child *needs* good mothering, but fathering is optional. It's good if a child grows up with a mother and father in the home, but if not, things will likely turn out OK. Dr. Warren Farrell has written a timely and critically important book on the importance of fathering for children, for men and women, and for society as a whole.

In *Father and Child Reunion: How to Bring the Dads We Need to the Children We Love* he offers detailed research on the problem and what we can do about it. According to Farrell, "One quarter of American children are living without their dads—that's 17 million children missing their dads, or never knowing what they're missing."

The consequence of the increasing loss of our fathering function is nothing short of a human tragedy. "Fatherlessness is the most harmful demographic trend of this generation," says Blankenhorn. "It is the leading cause of declining child well-being in our society. It is the engine driving our most urgent social problems, from crime to adolescent pregnancy to child sexual abuse to domestic violence against women."

Most agree that children need the active involvement of both parents if they are to grow up to be healthy, joyful adults. It is still generally assumed that if that is not possible, children are better off staying with their mothers. However, Farrell presents new evidence that suggests that if shared parent time isn't possible, children may be better off living with their dads, rather than with their moms.

"We prepared society for women entering the world of work by challenging ourselves to acknowledge that *sometimes* 'the best man for the job is a woman,'" says Farrell. "As we prepare men to enter the world of children, we need to be open to the possibility that *sometimes* 'the best mother for a child is the father.'"

The Shame of Our Bodies and the Wound of Circumcision

Marilyn Milos is a nurse and the mother of three circumcised boys. She was a student nurse in 1979 the day she first saw the operation performed. Here's how she described it in an interview:

> We students filed in the newborn nursery to find a baby strapped spread-eagle to a plastic board on a countertop across the room. He was struggling against his restraints—tugging, whimpering,

> and then crying helplessly. I finally asked the doctor if I could comfort the child. He soon relaxed under my touch and was momentarily quiet.
>
> The silence was soon broken by a piercing scream—the baby's reaction to having his foreskin pinched and crushed as the doctor attached the clamp to his penis. The shriek intensified when the doctor inserted an instrument between the foreskin and the glans [head of the penis], tearing the two structures apart. [They are normally attached to each other during infancy so the foreskin can protect the sensitive glans from urine and feces.] The baby started shaking his head back and forth—the only part of his body free to move—as the doctor used another clamp to crush the foreskin lengthwise, where he then cut. This made the opening of the foreskin large enough to insert a circumcision instrument, the device used to protect the glans from being severed during the surgery.
>
> The baby began to gasp and choke, breathless from his shrill, continuous screams. How could anyone say circumcision is painless when the suffering is so obvious?
>
> During the next stage of the surgery, the doctor crushed the foreskin against the circumcision instrument and then, finally, amputated it. The baby was limp, exhausted, spent.

For most of us born in the United States, this is an experience we share as males. We were too young to remember the event, but our bodies never forget.

As a Jewish male I was aware of the religious reasons given for circumcision. I was surprised, however, to find out that the original practice involved a symbolic removal of the tip of the foreskin. The more radical surgery practiced by modern Jews and the medical establishment, in which the entire foreskin is removed, is not in keeping with the original Jewish experience. Many modern Jews are replacing circumcision with an alternate ceremony of welcome that does not involve cutting of the foreskin.

If circumcision is so obviously painful and has no medical justification, why has it continued for so long?

We can get clues about the hidden agenda supporting circumcision if we understand why the practice began to spread in the United States in the late 1800s. Circumcision gained importance only after the medical profession, playing upon prevailing sexual anxieties, urged it as a "cure" for a long list of childhood diseases and disorders, including polio, tuberculosis, bed-wetting, and a new syndrome that appeared widely in the medical literature of the time—"masturbatory insanity."

Circumcision was then advocated along with a host of exceedingly harsh, pain-inducing devices and practices designed to thwart any vestige of genital pleasure in children and to ensure that they remained under parental control.

I found the religious roots and reasoning for circumcision by looking to my Jewish heritage. The 13th-century rabbi Moses Maimonides was more honest than almost anyone since in his reasons for supporting circumcision: "The bodily injury caused to that organ is exactly that which is desired, it does not interrupt any vital function, nor does it destroy the power of regeneration. Circumcision simply counteracts excessive lust; for there is no doubt that circumcision weakens the power of sexual excitement, and sometimes lessens the natural enjoyment."

We need to recognize that decreasing sexual pleasure and increasing sexual pain has a very useful purpose in "civilized" culture. It produces men who are numb, cut off from our feelings with a great deal of repressed rage. The real purpose of circumcising baby boys is to begin a process of taking the "wild" out of us.

Shame of all kinds serves the same purpose. Shame arises from loss, and it makes us more controllable by "civilization." The final step in the shaming process is that we forget the source of the shame.

The first step in healing is for us to remember what was done to us, feel the feelings we have so long repressed, and allow ourselves to grieve for what we have lost.

ACTION OPTION

Talk About the Shame in Your Life

Pick one of the areas of shame that you have experienced. Within the next week, share your thoughts and feelings with another man that you know. Ask him to tell you about his experiences.

PART III

The Men Alive Program for Physical Health

The Physical Health Questionnaire

Take the following questionnaire to see if your health practices are adding or subtracting from a long and healthy life. It's usually our bad habits that do us in. The more no answers you give to the questions the better.

1. Do you smoke or chew tobacco, or are you around a lot of secondhand smoke?
2. Do you eat butter, cream, sweets, and other saturated fats, as well as fried food like french fries?
3. Do you eat a lot of meat and a minimal amount of fresh fruits and vegetables?
4. Do you drink beer, wine, and/or liquor in excess (more than two drinks* per day)?
5. Do you drink more than 16 ounces of coffee a day?
6. Do you neglect to floss your teeth every day?
7. Do you engage in risky sexual (unprotected or promiscuous) or drug-related behavior that increases your risk of contracting HIV or viruses that can cause cancer?

---

* A standard drink is one 12-ounce bottle of beer, or wine cooler, one 5-ounce glass of wine, or 1.5 ounces of 80-proof distilled spirits.

8. Do you find you are often angry and irritable, even if you may not show it?
9. Do you often feel overstressed?
10. Do you avoid regular exercise?

ACTION OPTION

Change an Unhealthy Behavior

Look over your answers. For every no, give yourself a pat on the back for avoiding negative health habits. For every yes, think about any of these practices that you'd like to change. Pick one now and commit to changing one behavior this week.

CHAPTER 7

Food For Life: How to Really Eat Like a Man

> My doctor suggested a triple bypass . . . bars, restaurants and bakeries.
>
> —Dean Martin

MEN CONSUME MORE saturated fat and dietary cholesterol than women do. We are less likely than women to limit fat or red meat in our diets. Further, we eat fewer fruits and vegetables than women and consume less fiber. We more often skip breakfast and are less likely to limit sugar and sweet foods. We also drink far more coffee than women and are more likely to drink at least five cups each day.

When I was growing up we were taught that eating this way would make us big and strong. Now we know that it really makes us fat and sickly. Here are a few of the facts that have motivated me to change the way I eat:

- Next to cigarettes, diet is the number 1 killer of Americans, according to Dr. Michael McGinnis, director of the Office of Disease Prevention and Health Promotion at the U.S. Department of Health and Human Services.
- Risk of fatal prostate cancer for men who regularly consume meats, dairy products, and eggs is 360 percent higher than for men who use these products sparingly.
- The risk of death from heart attack for the average American man is 50 percent.

- On the other hand, the risk of death from heart attack for American men who consume no meat is 15 percent, and for men who consume no meat, dairy products, or eggs it is 4 percent.
- "If you're a meat eater, you are contributing to the destruction of the environment, whether you know it or not," says Neal Barnard, president of the Physicians Committee for Responsible Medicine. "Clearly the best thing you can do for the earth is to not support animal agriculture."
- According to Barnard, nearly 4 billion tons of topsoil are lost each year in the United States, chiefly because of overgrazing by livestock and unsustainable methods of growing feed.
- Each year 20 million people in the world die of malnutrition. If Americans reduced their intake of meat by 10 percent, the freed-up land, water, and energy could be used to provide an adequate diet for 60 million people.

We don't have to totally eliminate meat, dairy products, and eggs in order to reduce our risk of premature death and help the planet. We just need to learn to move in that direction. The bad news is that our modern way of life makes it difficult to eat well. The good news is that for over 99 percent of human history, some 4 million years, we practiced healthy eating habits. Our ancient memories still dwell within, reminding us of the kind of diet that is natural for humans.

What's Wrong With Eat, Drink, and Be Merry?

Many men I know seem to live by the adage "Eat, drink, and be merry—for tomorrow we die." It has a romantic ring to it that appeals to many of us. We picture a young officer fighting for his country. He lives fast and dies young. But in between he has a good life filled with all kinds of earthly pleasures.

For most of human history this wasn't a bad option. Life was short, old age was a time of frailty and disability, and death came quickly. In 1927 the average life span was around 45 years, and death was usually from acute disease. Hospitalization and/or dependency lasted for only days or, at most, weeks. In 1950 the average life span was about 58 years. Hospitalization and death usually took weeks or months. Under these circumstances, many men figured "Why not enjoy the life I have. If living well takes a few years off the end, who cares. At least I'll die happy."

But things have changed dramatically in the last 50 years. Now the average life span is approaching 80 years. Death from cancer, degenerative diseases, or immune deficiency usually takes years. The problem with "Eat, drink, and be merry" is that we're not likely to die "tomorrow." We're more likely to spend our last 20, 30, 40, or 50 years sick and miserable. That's not how I want my life to end—and I don't think you do, either.

Jonathan Swift wasn't too far off when he said that one of the best doctors in the world is "Doctor Diet." Medicine has come a long way since 1738, but Swift's dictum retains its truth. Learning about Doctor Diet is something most of us need to do.

Picture this: A man drives into the gas station and when approached by the attendant orders him to "fill it up" with milk and honey. "What did you say?" the attendant asked incredulously. "Milk and honey," the man repeats. "I like the sound of it. It looks good. That's what I grew up with, that's what I want in my tank."

The attendant can't believe what he is hearing. "But milk and honey won't work in your car. It isn't designed to run on milk and honey. It will ruin your engine. I've been trained to know what your car needs," he tells the man. "I can't give you something that is harmful."

The man drives away in a rage. He returns home, gets out a carton of milk and a jar of honey, and fills the gas tank to the brim. Satisfied, he goes inside and takes a nap, dreaming of childhood delights, of fast cars and fast girls. When he wakes up he dresses for a night on the town and puts on his new boots. He goes outside and slides into the front seat of his car and turns on the key. The engine coughs, sputters, and slowly dies.

The moral of the story is that regardless of childhood fun and fantasies, all things must be given the fuel they are made to run on or else they will die a premature and painful death. Most of us have little trouble understanding this when we think about our automobiles, but we have trouble applying it to what we put in our own bodies.

Over the years I've worked with men, I've realized that most of us know very little about good nutrition. "From early childhood, girls learn about food," says Dr. Royda Crose, author of *Why Women Live Longer Than Men.* "How to shop for it. How to prepare it. How it affects weight . . . Boys learn very little about the complexities of food. They just learn how to consume it." I believe that it's never too late to learn. So, come on guys, let's get started.

The Male American Diet (MAD) We Grew Up With

I grew up at a time when we knew a great deal less about health and diet than we do now. Now we recognize that eating large quantities of red meat and dairy products can lead to heart disease, diabetes, and cancer. When I was growing up, a big steak with a baked potato smothered in butter and sour cream were seen as health foods. Do you remember? I describe the Male American Diet as MAD because we now know that what we were taught was healthy was just the opposite.

Being a boy of slight build and short for my age, my mother encouraged me to eat meat in order to grow big and healthy. My stepfather, a strong, physical man, told me that eating a rare steak would make a man out of me. I believed him. *He* ate a lot of meat and *he* was strong. I came to love eating meat with a bright red center, the juices flowing when each piece is cut.

When we'd eat out, I'd order the biggest T-bone or porterhouse steak on the menu along with a big order of french fries (which also had to be healthy since they were a vegetable.) At home, french fries were usually reserved for a treat on the weekends, taking too long to make in the crunch times during the week. White rice was the complement to the beef during the week, which I usually covered with butter and whatever drippings were left from the hamburger or steak that was made.

I remember the TV ads for sides of beef with all kinds of luscious-sounding cuts that would be delivered to our home freezer prewrapped and ready to eat. Since my father left when I was quite young, my mother worked outside the home during most of my growing-up years. She'd come home tired, and I would often make a meal for both of us. I learned early how to make hamburgers and broil steaks. I would put potatoes in the oven to bake.

Sometimes I would remember that having some veggies was a good thing. I would usually cut a hunk of iceberg lettuce and cover it with a thick dressing. I figured that ketchup was also a good-enough vegetable to round out the diet. I felt proud to be able to cook a healthy meal at night.

In the morning my Mom had to get to work quickly, so making a hamburger with a leftover potato or rice seemed to be a good way to start the day. For lunch I would have some kind of meat sandwich. For most of my growing-up years I ate meat three times a day. I remember growing from being a skinny kid to one who had a belly on him by the time I was 9 or 10. I wasn't fat, just chunky. It never occurred to me or my mother that our diet was less than the best that money could buy.

I also learned that dairy products were good for you. "Drink your milk," my mother used to remind me. Eggs and cheese were also seen as healthy. Even ice cream was viewed as a health food. "It's made out of milk," my mother would say with a little catch in her voice that told me it wasn't as good as milk, but it was OK since it was made from milk.

In school I learned about the "Four Basic Food Groups," the two most important being meat and dairy products. I remember sitting in elementary school and listening to the teacher talk about good nutrition. She would bring out beautifully colored charts that had "scientific" information on nutrition and told us the importance of eating meat, drinking milk, and getting lots of protein.

I can still hear my teacher's refrain ringing in my ears: "Eat your meat and drink your milk so you will get enough protein and grow up to be strong." She would smile, and we would all smile back. I liked my teacher. She was young and pretty. I believed what she told me, and the pretty charts confirmed everything she was telling us.

No one, least of all an overworked teacher, questioned the truth of the information contained on those colorful charts. It didn't occur to us then to ask who promoted the idea that there were only four basic food groups and that good protein could only come from meat and dairy products. We never looked at the small print on the charts to see that they were being supplied by the National Egg Board, the National Dairy Council, and the National Livestock and Meat Board.

That doesn't necessarily make the information we received in school wrong, but it does tell us that those who were providing the information were clearly biased. They invested heavily in advertising to make us believe that we needed lots and lots of protein and that meat, eggs, and dairy products were the best sources of protein. The National Dairy Council is still the foremost supplier of "nutritional education" materials to classrooms in the United States. How helpful was their information?

Eating habits based on the Male American Diet are causing a host of diseases. Obviously you don't have to be male to suffer from eating this way. Women have learned to eat and die like men. But men seem to be more attached to eating in these unhealthy ways.

We Don't Need Meat (or a Lot of Animal Protein)

"The whole of man's hunting endeavor must be understood as a symbolic, cultural, and social activity," says social scientist Paul Shepard, author of *The Tender Carnivore and the Sacred Game.* "Though he is a highly capable social predator on large, dangerous mammals, he is singularly without the nutritional necessity of eating meat. He is a polished runner and stalker who eats meat as a sacrament."

For those of us who grew up in the meat-eating culture of the 1950s it is hard to believe that meat is not a necessity of life. Where would we get our protein?" we ask, fearful that we will die or, at the very least, lose our manly strength without it. We needn't worry. Even total vegetarians who don't eat any meat don't have to worry. We've learned a lot since I grew up that shows we needn't worry about getting our protein from meat.

"Research has discredited the idea that vegetable protein is incomplete and therefore less valuable than animal protein," says Andrew Weil, M.D., an expert on health and nutrition and the author of *Eating Well for Optimum Health.* "Not only can vegetarians survive and be healthy, studies consistently show them to be healthier and longer-lived than meat eaters."

Not only can we get healthy, complete protein from nonanimal sources, we don't need nearly as much protein as we think we do. "Protein needs are much lower than most people imagine," says Dr. Weil, "and the risk of protein deficiency for most of us is negligible." I would venture to say that there isn't one person who is reading this book that has to worry about protein deficiency. Even athletes and men engaged in heavy physical labor can get all they need from a diet rich in fruits, vegetables, cereals, and grains.

I was surprised to learn that even many world-class athletes seem to do quite well without eating meat. I remember watching Edwin Moses fly over the hurdles and win a gold medal in track and field in the Olympics. He went eight years without losing a race and was awarded the Sportsman of the Year award in 1984. I couldn't quite believe it when I found out that Edwin Moses is a vegetarian.

There are even weight lifters, guys who we would think would need to bulk up on beef, who seem to do quite well without it. Andreas Cahling is a Swedish bodybuilder who has won numerous international competitions. Competing at the highest levels in the world, Andreas remained a vegetarian throughout his career.

The Male American Diet Is Killing Us Slowly

The Male American Diet emphasizes meat, dairy products, saturated fats, and refined carbohydrates. We have all learned to love our hamburgers, ice cream, cheese, chips and dips, pizza, cakes, and cookies.

Dr. Weil says that a diet of this sort, though it will sustain life and growth, will also have tremendous consequences as we age. He says:

- It will increase the frequency of degenerative diseases.
- It will cause us to get these diseases at a younger age.
- It will accelerate the progression of these diseases and worsen their severity.
- It will certainly promote obesity, hypertension, coronary heart disease, and cancer and probably adversely affect liver, kidney, and brain function.

- By impairing immunity and the healing response, it should increase susceptibility to infection and toxic injury.
- By promoting inflammation, it may increase the incidence of arthritis, bursitis, tendinitis, and the general aches and pains of aging.
- It might make people less energetic and worsen their moods.

ACTION OPTION

Change the Male American Diet

Write a list of the Male American Diet foods you commonly eat. Put a star next to the ones you know are the worst for you. Make a decision to eliminate those foods from your diet for the next month. Substitute the foods you are giving up with healthy alternatives.

For instance, if you are giving up ice cream, you may want to substitute nonfat frozen yogurt. If you are giving up hamburger, you may want to substitute a veggie burger (they are a lot tastier than you might imagine).

The Six Best Diets In the World

A simple way of finding the best diets is to look at all the characteristics of the Deadly Diet and then look in the opposite direction. I have found that a "stay-away" diet doesn't work well because we are constantly repeating in our minds, "I shouldn't eat ________" which reinforces our focus on what is *not* good for us. I believe a better approach is to put our attention on a way of eating that is the most life enhancing.

In his book *Eating Well for Optimum Health,* Dr. Andrew Weil has put together the six best diets from leading experts throughout the world. He also includes the advantages and disadvantages of each. The diets he discusses are the following:

1. *The Paleolithic Diet.* This emphasizes lean meat from wild game, fish, wild fruits, nuts, tubers, and some vegetables.

2. *The Raw Food Diet.* This takes us back to a time in our historical past before we cooked our food. It emphasizes uncooked fruits, vegetables, seeds, nuts, and lots of fiber.

3. *The Traditional Japanese Diet.* This emphasizes vegetables, both raw and cooked, fresh fish, and rice. Until recently, the Japanese were the healthiest people on the planet. They are still the longest-lived people, with men living on average 77.2 years and women 84.1 years. The recent change for the worse seems to be due to a shift to eating a more Western diet.

4. *The "Asian Diet."* There are many healthy Asian diets emphasizing cuisine from different countries and regions. They all share an emphasis on eating lots of fruits and vegetables, less milk and meat, and more fish than our Western diet, and use tea as the main beverage.

5. *The Vegan Diet.* With this diet we eat no animal foods—including milk, dairy products, eggs, or flesh foods. It emphasizes vegetables, fruits, grains, and legumes.

6. *The Mediterranean Diet.* This diet draws on the cuisines of Spain, southern France, Italy, Greece, Crete, and parts of the Middle East. It emphasizes breads, pasta, rice, and other grains. It also includes lots of fruits, fish, beans, legumes, nuts, and vegetables. Meat is not emphasized.

Dr. Weil particularly likes the Mediterranean Diet. He feels it conforms to most of the principles of healthy nutrition. "It is a style of eating that I like very much," he says, "and one associated with much lower incidence of obesity, cardiovascular disease, and cancer than in most of Europe and the Americas."

I have found that there is no right or wrong diet. We can even indulge ourselves from time to time. With so much healthy and tasty food to choose from, there really is no excuse for putting unhealthy things into our bodies. We can also mix and match items from the healthy diets, which is what I do.

I don't have the knowledge or the patience to prepare good Asian food, but I love to go out to restaurants that specialize in Japanese, Chinese, Indian, or Thai cuisine. At home I eat mostly vegetarian food with lots of good veggies and fruits, and some good fish once in awhile. You will find your own favorite way of eating. Here are some guiding principles that I have found to be helpful.

The 12 Principles for Healthy Eating

1. Keep it simple.

Do you get as confused as I do about all the claims and counter claims of what is the best diet? We hear about the High Protein-Low Carbohydrate diet, the High Carbohydrate-Low Protein, the Blood Type diet, and a hundred more. This expert disagrees with that expert. Who has time to try and figure it all out? I don't and I don't think you do either. Just remember that it doesn't take much to begin improving on what and how we eat. If you want to delve into more depth, I will provide resources at the end of the book.

2. Eating should be pleasurable.

Those of us who grew up on hamburgers and french fries also grew up believing that eating health food was about as pleasurable as eating grass. I remember hearing the "health nuts" of the 1950s talk about eating wheat grass, juicing carrots, and subsisting on cabbage and grapefruit.

The opposite of the Male American Diet is not the Inedible and Boring Diet. We can, and should, have food that gives us pleasure. This is particularly important as we get older. "I like food," says Dr. Weil. "I experience pleasure from eating, and I am unwilling to sacrifice that experience in a quest for better health. . . . My conviction is that healthy food and delicious food are not mutually exclusive; the concept of 'eating well' must embrace both the health-promoting and pleasure-giving aspects of food." I couldn't agree more.

3. Eating well and getting enough exercise go together.

Not only are we designed to eat a diet rich in fruits, vegetables, and complex carbohydrates, but we are designed to combine food and exercise. Think about it. Whether hunting or gathering, our ancestors had to move to get the food that they ate each day. Exercise and eating are opposite sides of the same coin. In order to remain healthy and live long and well, we need to combine the two.

There is a simple formula for keeping our weight in the healthy range. We must expend as much energy as we take in. In our hunter-gatherer past, that was built into the process. If we didn't move, we didn't eat. The more we ate the more active we had to be. Now we can eat a lot without expending much energy. If we are gaining more weight as we age, we can be sure that we need to eat fewer calories and increase our exercise program.

4. Variety is the spice of life.

There is so much good, healthy food available to most of us that we don't have to be content with eating the same old thing. We need to get creative, try different foods, and give our taste buds a chance to find a variety of new foods that we really like.

5. Get fresh with your fruits and vegetables.

The more fresh food we eat, the better. The more we can eat fruits and vegetables the better. When I go to the market I head for the produce section. Filling up our shopping cart in this section means good health and lower cost. If the produce section looks like foreign territory to you, try starting with canned and frozen foods and add more fresh foods as you go along.

6. Fat is not bad. We need the right amount and the right kinds.

For many people, cutting down on fats has become an obsession. Fat is seen as a kind of bogeyman that is out to kill us, yet is so seductive we can't seem to stay away from him. The truth is that fat is essential for life. Among other things, you couldn't absorb vitamins A, D, and E without fat.

Another truth that most of us experience every day is that while we might hate fat around the waist, we love it in our mouths.

There is a simple reason why we like to eat cake, chocolate chip cookies, potato chips, pizza, steak, french fries—to name a few of my favorites over the years. Fat tastes good. Chocolate is appealing to many of us, in part, because of the sensuous feeling left in your mouth by the cocoa butter it contains.

So don't run away from fat; embrace it. Reduce saturated fat by eating less butter, fatty meats, cream, cheese, and other full-fat dairy products and by eating more fish, fortified eggs, soybeans, olive oil, canola oil, flaxseed oil, and nuts. Do your best to stay away from fried foods.

7. We don't have to worry about getting enough protein. We need the right kind.

We should eat more vegetable protein, especially from beans. Soybeans and soy products are particularly good. They come in a great variety. It took me awhile to get used to soy products, but now I love them. We should eat less animal protein. Fish, such as wild Alaskan salmon, are a good source of protein and other nutrients, as are reduced-fat dairy products. If you like meat, try eating bison or wild game. If you like chicken, get drug- and hormone-free, free-range chicken, favor the white meat, and remove the skin before cooking. If you eat eggs, use omega-3-fortified, organically raised eggs from free-range chickens. Turkey is a good source of protein. Get the hormone-free, free-range variety. You don't even have to wait for Christmas or Thanksgiving.

8. Eat more complex carbohydrates with a low glycemic index.

Growing up, I believed that next to protein, carbohydrates were the best nutrients we could eat. Bread was, after all, the staff of life. I thought all carbohydrates were the same. They are not. Carbohydrates are found naturally in foods in two forms: simple and complex.

We should eat more foods containing complex carbohydrates, including fruits like apples and oranges, and starches and vegetables like peas, potatoes, beans, pasta, and corn. We should eat fewer foods containing simple carbohydrates like sugar, corn syrup, milk, and fruit juices.

Once I got my list of complex carbohydrates I thought I was home free, until I learned that even many complex carbohydrates have a high glycemic index (GI)—which means they are broken down more quickly to simple carbohydrates and, if not needed by the body for quick energy, can turn into fat.

Here are some popular foods containing complex carbohydrates with a high glycemic index (pure glucose is 100). Don't eat too many of these.

- White rice—72
- White bread—70
- Baked potatoes—93
- Bagels—72
- Cornflakes—84

Popular complex carbohydrate foods with lower glycemic indices include:

- Brown rice—55
- Sourdough bread or pumpernickel bread—52
- Sweet potatoes—54
- Soybeans—18

- Corn—55
- Spaghetti—43

9. Stay regular; eat fiber.

If you've gotten this far with me, you will find this principle simple to follow. All animal products—including meat, poultry, dairy products, eggs, fish, and shellfish—contain no fiber. All unprocessed plant foods are high in dietary fiber. You do the math.

10. Take a few supplements.

Eating our fruits and veggies will take us a long way to getting the vitamins and minerals we need. But most of us wonder if we should take supplements, and if so what kinds. We are bombarded with a huge array of promises that if we take the right kinds of supplements we will live longer and better. I recently held one bottle that says it contains "the world's best nutritional supplement." It tells me it has a "super antioxidant-rich formula." Sound familiar?

In following our first principle, let's keep it simple. I suggest you take the following:

- Aspirin, 165 milligrams (mg), which is half of a regular tablet (it thins the blood and protects us against the risk of a heart attack)
- Vitamin B complex, which contains at least 400 micrograms (mcg) of folic acid as well as vitamins B_6, 50 mg and B_{12}, 800 mcg
- Vitamin C, 100 mg twice a day (recent research shows you don't need any more than that—your body will just flush it out)
- Mixed carotenoids, 25,000 international units (IU)
- Calcium, 1,200 to 1,500 mg
- Natural vitamin E, 400 to 800 mg (the higher number if we are over 55)
- Selenium, 200 mcg of a yeast-bound form

11. Protect Your Prostate.

For some reason our prostate gland often grows larger as we age and puts pressure on the bladder. Our "busy bladder" can cause us to wake up numerous times at night and force us to stay close to a bathroom during the day. I've had to think of driving long distances in terms of rest room availability or where I can find privacy along the highway.

There are a number of things we can do to prevent or reduce the effects of these problems.

- Decrease intake of animal foods and saturated fat.
- Eat soy foods regularly.
- Eat plenty of fresh fruits and vegetables, including cooked tomatoes (in tomato sauce made with olive oil, for example).
- Eat whole grains, nuts, and seeds, especially raw (or freshly toasted) pumpkin seeds.
- Take an extract of saw palmetto (it's made from the berries of a plant native to the American Southeast and has been shown to reduce the size of the prostate in the vast majority of men). I recommend you take 160 mg twice a day and that you use a product that contains at least 85 percent of the active fatty acids.

12. Drink the Big Three: water, green tea, and red wine.

All of us should drink more water. I recommend six to eight glasses a day. This isn't easy in the best of circumstances, but when we have to pee frequently, it can be even more difficult. Give it your best shot.

Green tea is a soothing beverage and contains antioxidants that have been shown to prevent disease.

If you drink alcohol, drink red wine. The red pigments have antioxidants that are helpful. Just remember it's the "red," not the alcohol, that is healthy. You can get the same benefits from drinking red grape juice or eating plenty of red or purple fruits. The pigments in them protect our hearts, lungs, and blood vessels from degenerative changes.

ACTION OPTION

Add Healthy Foods

Pick one item that you believe would benefit your health. Implement it some time this week. Add another item each week for the next month. Keep track of how you feel and consider adding new ones when you are ready.

Why Is It So Hard to Eat Well even When We Know the Truth?

Although I learn a bit more about nutrition each day, most of this information I have known for a long time. It seems so simple. Stay away from the foods listed on the Deadly Diet and find healthy alternatives from a wide assortment of Good Diet choices.

Yet I have found it devilishly difficult to consistently follow the program that I have outlined for you above. I'll do fine for awhile, then slip back into old patterns. At times I have felt like giving up. I have recently come to recognize the power of the forces that work against us. With this added knowledge we can devise a program that will make it easier for all of us to be successful.

1. Our evolutionary needs work against us.

Remember we have a 4 million year old heritage in which fats and sweets were scarce and hard to come by. Our ancestors had a built-in body mechanism that said in effect, "If you see or hear of any sweet or high fat foods, pursue them without delay, and eat as much as you can." Most of us have inherited a "fat tooth" along with a "sweet tooth" for the same evolutionary reasons. Eating as much as we could get made good sense during our evolutionary past. If we do the same thing now it can be deadly.

Our minds and bodies have not had enough time to adapt to this new environment. They are still built for the past: "Look for it, eat it, and keep eating it" remains the default setting. It's no wonder we have a difficult time controlling our sweet tooth and fat tooth. They have 4 million years of weight on their side.

Here's what we can do: We need a strong counterweight, something to oppose the immediate desire to eat all those goodies. This means consciously limiting ourselves. Here's what I do. I pretend that I still live in a world where fats and sweets are scarce. I never eat more than one goodie a month. I stay away from places where I might run into them more often, like pizza and ice cream parlors. If I know I'm going to a place where goodies will be served, I bring something healthy to eat instead.

2. Our family food experiences work against us.

Many of us were raised at a time when fats and sweets were seen as OK, if not health foods. Whether we liked our family or not, the foods from our childhood have a strong physical, emotional, and sensous impact on us, long after we leave home.

I can still hear the hamburgers sizzling in the frying pans. I can feel the stacks of buttery toast that I dipped into my cocoa. I can smell the grilled cheese sandwiches as I took my first bite. I can see the hot fudge sundaes and banana splits that I would get regularly at Curry's ice cream parlor.

In addition to the general goodies that we grew up with, there were also "reward" and "comfort" foods. Remember those? If you're a good boy, Mommy or Daddy will buy you ——— (fill in the blank). For me, it was always ice cream. The better I'd been, the bigger the treat. What was your reward food?

Most of us also had comfort foods that we ate to cheer us up when we were sad. Mine were pastries. When I felt down I would crave cinnamon rolls. I would go to the bakery, intent on buying one, but would often buy six. There were many times that I'd eat them all and go back for another half dozen.

Here's what we can do: The old experiences that influence our eating are often unconscious. The best way to become a master of your eating habits is to become aware of what influences you. What are your memories? If you're like me, they may have been long forgotten but still are a powerful influence on what and how we eat. To give us a chance to resist the temptations that come from our family background, we need a strategy.

I have found it helpful to look back and find the healthy foods that I *did* eat growing up, even if they are few and far between. I loved corn on the cob and rarely ate it with butter. I ate spinach because I wanted to grow up to be strong like Popeye. I drank V-8 juice because I like to be different.

We also need to find new reward and comfort foods. For comfort I still like to go to the bakery. But now I get healthy, thick-crusted, fresh-baked bread, which I love and eat right out of the oven.

3. Eating out works against us.

We've come a long way since we hunted and gathered, cooked, and ate our own food. But even in my youth there was a time that my parents raised chickens for their eggs and meat, and we also had a small vegetable garden. Although, as I see now, my diet had some severe limitations, we ate at home most of the time.

But now with many of us, both husband and wife, working long hours, we eat more and more of our meals away from home. In 1978, we got 18 percent of our calories from food eaten away from home. Now it's almost twice that much and still climbing. Although we may try to eat healthy when we eat out, we are fighting an uphill battle.

"Everything about restaurants encourages overeating," says Susan Roberts, a nutrition researcher from Tufts University in Medford, Massachusetts. "The food is high in fat and is calorie-dense, so it tastes good and you eat it so quickly that you're done before you start to feel full."

When we eat bulky, high-fiber foods like vegetables, fruits, and whole grains, we get fewer calories per swallow, so there's more time for the stretch receptors in our stomachs to make us feel full. That's why we can eat a lot and not feel full at first. Later, after we've left the restaurant, we notice that we feel stuffed. After awhile we get used to that stuffed feeling, and we don't feel like we've had a complete meal until we know we are stuffed.

Here's what we can do: Clearly we can eat out less often. But for many of us, we need quick meals or we wouldn't have meals at all. What I often do is to eat a snack, like a few carrot sticks, celery, or raisins, *before* I go to the restaurant. When I'm not so hungry I don't order as much, eat as fast, or eat so much. We can also pick restaurants with simple, healthy food. That's one of the reasons I like going to Asian restaurants.

Find a healthy restaurant that makes the dining experience super-enjoyable. My current favorite is a Chinese restaurant, where they have come to know me and treat me like one of the family. They will make anything I want and do it without oil. I'm particularly fond of the eggplant.

I find I have to avoid any restaurant that has a buffet. There's so much to choose from that I always eat too much, even if it's healthy food. I can't seem to leave until I've gotten my money's worth, even if it means eating more than I want.

4. Modern advertising works against us.

Spend a day seeing how many food ads you see in a 16-hour period. You probably already know that you are being bombarded, but you will still be surprised by the extent of the ads. Look at what we get on the TV, on billboards, in our magazines and newspapers, on the radio, and over the Internet.

"Don't just stand there! Eat something!" urge the ads for granola bars at bus stops. Most of what we are being asked to eat are generally things that are bad for us. Restaurant ads have topped the $3 billion a year mark. Candy and snack ads are over $1 billion a year. Soft drinks are close to a billion and beer ads are everywhere.

If we didn't learn to eat poorly at home, we are now learning in our schools. Advertisers have become much more sophisticated than when I was growing up. Along with the nicely colored charts telling the kids to eat more meat, eggs, and dairy products, we now have TV in the classrooms. More than 12,000 classes subscribe to Channel One, a daily commercial television news program broadcast by satellite. "These schools force their children to sit and watch commercials for fast foods and soft drinks, the very kinds of foods that are making them fatter," says Gary Ruskin, director of Commercial Alert, a nonprofit group in Washington, D.C., that opposes excesses in commercialism, advertising, and marketing.

Here's what we can do: It's hard to stay away from advertising in today's world. But we can reduce its effect just by being aware of what the goal is. Notice that we are not bombarded by ads for fruits and vegetables. Advertisers play on our evolutionary hunger for fats and sweets.

Though difficult, we can "just say no." Fats and sweets are as addictive (maybe even more so) than marijuana or cocaine. However, willpower is not enough. We have to fill ourselves up with the good stuff so that there isn't so much room for the bad stuff. Eat well, and you will be less influenced by the marketing madness that is meant to hook you.

For clients who have had trouble with alcohol, I recommend that they stay out of bars. For all of us who want to keep from being victimized by advertising, I recommend that we stay away from it as much as we can. I rarely watch commercial TV in the evening. That's my most vulnerable time to go "snacking" for something to eat. It's also prime time for the advertisers. If I do watch, I immediately turn the sound off as soon as a commercial comes on and get away from the TV until the show I'm watching returns.

Do these things seem extreme to you? They did to me, too. But I realized that I needed extreme measures to counter the powerful weight of our evolutionary heritage, our childhood hungers, our mobile lifestyle, and the pressures of advertising.

Eat well—and you'll live well.

CHAPTER 8

Testosterone and Other Male Hormones: What We Need to Know

It seems certain that testosterone is a hormone whose time has finally come.

—Malcolm Carruthers, M.D.

INTERESTINGLY, it was my wife, Carlin, who first got me thinking about the importance of male hormones. I had watched her progress over the years as she went through the menopause passage. I tried to be supportive, and I think I was most of the time. What would really throw me off were her sudden physical and emotional changes that didn't seem to have anything to do with what was going on in the "real world."

She would turn red and break out into a sweat for no apparent reason. We'd be driving home late after a movie. I'd want to turn the heater on to warm up the car. She wanted to open the window to "get some air circulating."

One minute she'd be happily "normal," the next minute she'd be withdrawn and sullen. Weeks would go by when I couldn't do anything right around her. Everything I did seemed to annoy her. Nearly every day she'd tell me, with barely concealed anger, that I'd left the dishes out. Or I hadn't put the food in the refrigerator. Or I had put the food away, but I hadn't wrapped the potatoes properly.

Even though I knew intellectually that there was a real world changing inside her, I still had a difficult time accepting that her moods and behavior could be so influenced by her hormones. She never used her hormones as an excuse for her behavior. I think she was sensitive to all the times when women have been labeled and excluded from social life because they were "hormonal."

Carlin began her "change of life" in her early 40s and didn't come through completely until her mid to late 50s. During that time it was her mood swings, lack of sexual desire, and irritability that bothered me the most. The change took much longer than I had ever thought and was difficult on both of us. It never occurred to me that I might be going through something similar.

Carlin is five and a half years older than I am, and she came through menopause while I was still at the height of andropause. While she was in the midst of the change it was easy for me to blame our marital ups and downs, fights, and unhappy sex life on her. But when the same problems remained after she no longer had a role to play I had to begin to look at myself.

Carlin forced me to. At first she was soft and gentle about it: "Hey, hon, maybe you're going through some kind of hormonal change, too." Sometimes I'd roll my eyes and shake my head, as if to say, "Give me a break. You're the one who has hormonal fluctuations, always have and probably always will." At other times, I'd smile sweetly and tell her, "Maybe you're right dear." Then I'd go up to my office and try and forget the whole thing.

But our hormones have a way of not letting us forget that they are there. Remember adolescence? I know if you're like me, that's a time you'd as soon forget. Remember the erections that would seem to pop up unbidden, just at the worst time?

I'd get called on to recite something in front of the class and have to keep my notebook placed strategically in front of my lap in order maintain some semblance of dignity. When the bell would ring and it was time to move to my next class, I'd often have to sit for what seemed like an eternity pretending to gather my things while thinking of iceboxes and dead bodies in the hopes that my arousal would subside enough to allow me to walk.

Then there were the constant reminders from older boys who seemed bent on tormenting me. When I'd be trying to stay cool and collected talking to Nancy, some guy would stroll by and whisper loud enough for everyone to hear, "Hey, Diamond, I'm wise to the rise in your Levis." And God forbid that I would ever get caught with a hand in my pants pocket: "What ya doin', playin' pocket pool?"

Maybe it's our reluctance to recall the pain and shame of adolescence that keeps us from wanting to recognize the hormonal changes that occur as we age. The truth is that hormones are a critical part of what makes us human. They are present throughout our lives and often come to our attention during transition periods like adolescence and andropause.

I often describe andropause as like adolescence in reverse. During adolescence hormones are increasing, and during andropause they are decreasing. In many ways the two stages of life are similar. Both involve tremendous hormonal shifts. During adolescence the shift is very rapid and dramatic. During andropause the shift is slower, yet the changes that occur can be just as difficult to deal with and just as troublesome.

What Are Hormones and Why Should We Care?

We now know much more about hormones and the male body. But for most men, hormones are still a mystery.

Hormones are one of the body's great communication networks; the others are the nervous and immune systems. A hormone molecule, released by one of about a dozen glands, travels through the blood until it reaches a cell with a receptor that it fits. Then, like a key in a lock, the molecule attaches to the receptor and sends a signal inside the cell. The signal may tell the cell to produce a certain protein or to multiply.

Hormones are involved in just about every biological process: immune function, reproduction, growth, even controlling other hormones. They can work at astonishingly small concentrations—in parts per billion or trillion. Humans have about 50 different known hormones.

Some hormones are relatively well known, such as testosterone, estrogen, and progesterone. Others are less well known, such as human growth hormone (HGH), melatonin, DHEA (dehydroepiandrosterone), and thyroid hormone. Still others are known only to a few, such as oxytocin, vasopressin, and pregnenolone. Yet all are vitally important to the functioning of the human body.

Many scientists now believe that it is the loss of hormones throughout the years that is the key to many of the unpleasant symptoms of aging. They also feel, as you will see later in this chapter, that replacing missing hormones is the key to staying sexy and healthy throughout your life.

Pheromones: The Essence of Male and Female Attraction

Pheromones are substances that many animals, including humans, give off into the air and are picked up by others of the same species. These olfactory essences are instrumental in bringing males and females together and influencing behaviors, including sexual attraction and readiness.

Pheromones are very similar to hormones. Like hormones, pheromones are substances that are produced in the glands of the body. Like hormones, they travel some distance from their origins to act within the glands in the body. The difference between hormones and pheromones is this: whereas hormones exert their effects *within* one body, pheromones exert their effects *between* two or more different bodies.

For some time now scientists have known that when women live in close proximity, such as in a college dormitories, their menstrual cycles become more similar as time goes on. Recently scientists have found that it is pheromones that bring about this synchronicity.

In 1986 Dr. Winnifred Çutler and her colleagues at the University of Pennsylvania demonstrated that these essences were present in humans, and that they could be captured and preserved for use in the future. "My colleagues and I had demonstrated," said Cuttler, "that it was possible to bottle the essences of men and women, freeze them for a year, then thaw them, apply them to the skin under the nose somewhat like perfume, and change the endocrine milieu of the women who received them."

Men and women seem to have a natural essence that attracts us to each other. However, as we age our pheromones decrease, along with our sensitivity to these vital substances. As we shall see later in this chapter, it is possible to replace our flagging pheromones as well as our decreasing hormones and keep our attraction juices flowing even as we age.

Why Men Have "Female" Hormones and Women Have "Male" Hormones

When we think of female hormones we often think of estrogen, and when we think of male hormones we often think of testosterone. But testosterone isn't the only hormone that is of importance to men. Estrogen is also vital to male well-being and happiness. We know that although men have more testosterone than women and women have more estrogen than men, both hormones are present in males and females.

Estrogen in the male bloodstream may account for his desire, not just for sex, but for love and intimacy. Estrogen promotes receptivity and touching, qualities that both men and women value.

Many Americans remember the outpouring of response when Ann Landers asked whether women preferred hugging and cuddling "to the act itself." Over 20,000 women responded. Most said they preferred loving touch to sexual intercourse.

It would have been interesting if Ann Landers could have gotten an honest response from men to the same question. Contrary to the myth that all men want is sex, most of us, particularly as we get older, want and need to touch and be touched. There are times we need sensual and emotional intimacy even more than sexual connection.

When my wife, Carlin, was at the height of her menopause and we were the most distant, I greatly missed our sex life. But even more than sex, I missed the loving touch that usually accompanied it.

ACTION OPTION

Talk About Menopause

Talk to a woman you know who is going through menopause. Ask her to tell you about the physical, emotional, and hormonal changes she has noticed. Talk about your own change of life. Each of you write out a few pages on your experiences and compare notes.

Just as women have considerably less testosterone than men throughout most of their lives, men have considerably less estrogen. Just as recent research has shown the importance of testosterone in the lives of women, we are beginning to recognize that estrogen (as well as other hormones) are important to the lives of men. We can't call estrogen the female hormone and testosterone the male hormone.

Women are beginning to discover that they not only lose estrogen as they age, but also experience decreasing levels of testosterone. Many women have been told that taking estrogen and progesterone will help them as they age. Until recently few were told about the value of testosterone.

Hormonal Shifts and Sexual Cycles: Men Have Them, Too

Although most of us now accept that women and men have "male" and "female" hormones, it is more difficult to accept that men also have hormonal cycles. Yet, according to endocrinologist Dr. Estelle Ramey, a professor at Georgetown University Medical School, we most certainly do. "The evidence of them may be less dramatic," says Dr. Ramey, "but the monthly changes are no less real." But if men do have hormonal cycles, why don't we recognize them or talk about them?

Dr. Ramey believes it is because men respond to their cycles in a way that is a function of their "culturally acquired self-image. They deny them." This denial is the main reason she feels the largely male scientific and medical communities have taken so long to study andropause.

Men who are out of touch with our body rhythms, afraid that cycles are feminine and hence to be avoided at all costs, are unlikely to be aware of the subtle changes in our internal worlds.

Dr. Cutler is another modern researcher who has found a significant relationship between male sexuality and hormone changes. Like many women I have talked to, she began to recognize the hormonal patterns in men after studying shifts in women's cycles. For over 30 years her research has addressed the nature of the reproductive system of men and women, the effects of male and female hormones, the sexual and behavioral implications of hormones, and the changes in men and women as they age.

It has only been in recent years that we have greatly expanded our understanding of the hormonal changes men experience throughout our lives and how they change as we age.

Like the rotation of the earth and the ebb and flow of the tides, many of our hormones rise and fall within our bodies in cycles. A cycle might last a few minutes, a day, a week, a month, a season, a year, or a lifetime. There are also cycles within cycles.

We know, for instance, that a man's testosterone will fluctuate four or five times an hour. There is also research that shows that men think about sex, on average, four or five times an hour. Is this a coincidence or hormonal fact of life? Some researchers believe that as we age our hormonal cycles change.

ACTION OPTION

Compare Sexuality in Adolescence and Middlescence

Find a quiet spot where you will not be disturbed. Write down the memories you have of your sexual desires during adolescence. Pay particular attention to surges of sexual desire that would occur during each hour, day, and month. Now write down your memories of your sexual ups and downs in your middle years, between 40 and 55. Compare the two times of life and notice how you feel about the changes you are experiencing now.

If a young man, for instance, has blood taken from his arm six times a day starting in the early morning and continuing every four hours thereafter, lab results will tend to show a rhythmic rise and fall of testosterone reflecting the time of the day.

When he goes to sleep, his hormone levels will start rising hour by hour until, by the time he wakes, his testosterone levels will be at their highest. By late morning his levels are likely to level off and begin to decline. By late afternoon his testosterone will usually be at its lowest ebb.

Men's hormones also cycle throughout the year. In studies conducted in the United States, France, and Australia it was found that men secrete their highest levels of sex hormones in October and their lowest levels in April. There was a 16 percent increase in testosterone levels from April to October and a 22 percent decline from October to the next April. Interestingly, although Australia is in its springtime when France and the United States are in their autumn, men in all three parts of the world showed a similar pattern of peaks in October and valleys in April.

Men also have monthly hormonal cycles, though there are some interesting differences and similarities between women's and men's cycles. Women's monthly cycles are more predictable and synchronous.

A study of 20 young men showed that the majority had a discernible cycle of testosterone with regularly repeating rises and falls, but each man who did show a cycle had one unique to himself and different from the others.

Premenstrual syndrome (PMS), long associated with women, may be a fact of life for men as well. "One of the most misleading consequences of the popular focus on Premenstrual Syndrome," says psychologist Carol Tavris, "is that it omits men as a comparison group."

In one study, when men were given the same checklists of symptoms from a typical PMS questionnaire—omitting the female-specific symptoms, such as breast tenderness—men report having as many symptoms as women. We report having such symptoms as a decrease or an increase of energy, irritability and other negative moods, back pain, sleeplessness, headaches, and confusion. We also report noticing these changes at certain times of the month.

Psychologist Jessica McFarlane and her associates, who conducted the study, conclude that "women are not 'moodier' than the men; their moods were not less stable within a day or from day-to-day. Evidence of weekday mood cycles in both sexes suggests that treating emotional fluctuations as unhealthy symptoms, and assuming that only women usually manifest them, is misleading."

ACTION OPTION:

Observe Your Moods, Sexuality, and Energy

If you have a partner with whom you live, talk to your partner about what he or she observes about your feelings and behavior. See if your partner notices changes in your mood, sexuality, or energy at different times of the month. Write down your partner's observations. Write down what you notice about changes in yourself.

The final hormonal cycle that men must deal with, and one that is influenced by all the other shifts, involves the drop in hormone levels that occurs in midlife. As we saw in chapter 3, this cycle is associated with andropause. We are learning more and more about the way in which our changing hormone levels affect us physically, emotionally, and sexually.

After examining the research, interviewing hundreds of men, and observing my own changes hourly, daily, monthly, yearly, and at midlife, I am convinced that men experience significant hormonal changes throughout our lives. It is also clear to me that these changes greatly influence our health and well-being.

Perhaps the proverbial battle of the sexes would produce fewer casualties if men and women recognized how similar they were and how much our physical and emotional health is influenced by our hormones.

Hormone Replacement for Men?

There are an increasing number of health care professionals that believe that humans are on the brink of finding the key to the "fountain of youth." Many believe that we may soon be able to extend our healthy years beyond anything many of us have dreamed of achieving.

Welcome to what William Regelson, M.D., one of its major proponents, calls the "Superhormone Revolution": "When taken in combinations tailored to your particular needs, the superhormones are the juggernaut against the aging process." So what are these superhormones? Regelson believes there are eight of them: DHEA, pregnenolone, thyroid hormone, human growth hormone, melatonin, estrogen, progesterone, and testosterone.

Proponents of this antiaging medicine approach to health believe that aging itself is a disease that can be overcome. They believe that youthful resilience can be maintained throughout life and that hormone replacement therapy is the key to keeping our youthful appearance, abilities, and resiliency.

The desire to stay young forever is one that humans have sought for a long time. It seems now to be driven by the 76 million baby boomers and new technologies that offer the hope of eternal youth. I have found that it is us men who are particularly intrigued by notion of keeping our youthful vitality and sexuality as we age.

On the September 16, 1996, cover of *Newsweek* magazine the title read: "'Super-Hormone' Therapy: Can It Keep Men Young?" Inside we see a picture of the young man we once were (or wish we were) at 25, with wavy blond hair, strong muscles, rock hard abs, and a sexy, confident look in his eyes. We also see a balding, middle-aged guy with flabby arms and a bulging gut. He has a worried look on his face and stares longingly at the young man from his youth.

If the picture leaves any doubt about our decline, there is a "helpful" chart that details our loss of brain function, hair, vision, heart response, hearing, aerobic endurance and lung power, lean bodies, muscle and bone strength, and, of course, erections and frequency of sex.

The caption under Dr. Regelson's picture says this: "Time in a bottle: With the right chemical cocktail of super-hormones no one has to get old at all. It is possible to slow and even reverse the aging process." Who in his right mind wouldn't be interested in that?

The truth is that if the superhormones delivered on all their promises, we would *all* sign up to receive our youth-producing cocktail. Although proponents offer a wonderful view of the future of hormone therapy they rarely talk about the current state of the art or the possible downside of hormone treatments.

For instance, DHEA is untested in long-term clinical trails and its strength and purity are not regulated. Melatonin is unregulated and largely untested; grogginess or mild depression are reported side effects. Both these powerful hormones can be gotten in most health food stores.

I even found them being sold at my corner gas station. I don't know about you, but I'm more than a little suspicious when I hear about the latest wonder drug that can do miraculous things for my body. I'm even more suspicious when I can purchase some from the clerk at my local fill-'em-up-and-go gas station.

On the cover of the book *Grow Young with HGH,* by Dr. Ronald Klatz, we are told that HGH (human growth hormone) will help us "lose fat, build muscle, reverse the effects of aging, strengthen the immune system, lower our blood pressure and cholesterol, and improve sexual performance." We are not told that there have not been long-term studies that demonstrate its value. Nor are we told that there are potential dangers, including diabetes and enlarging bones and internal organs.

Although hormones do offer a promise for a positive future, I don't believe that many of them have yet proven their efficacy. Though some of the recent findings on their value are provocative, I'm not convinced that taking these superhormones will solve all our problems. We'd all like to be handsome, strong, vital, and sexy in our 20s and keep it up into our 50s, 60s, 70s, and beyond.

As I've already told you, hormonal health is only part of what we need. We need to focus as well on the physical, nutritional, mental, interpersonal, social, and spiritual aspects of health. Yet hormones *are* important. There is one hormone that is vital to men's health that I believe has a long enough history of use to have proven its value. This hormone is testosterone.

I Want Testosterone

Henry is a 56-year-old man, recently married for the third time. He came to our clinic because he felt something was wrong and he was concerned he wouldn't be able to keep up with his younger wife. He was overweight, out of shape, drank too much, and was depressed. He had recently retired from a high-stress job and felt at loose ends. He had no idea what he wanted to do with the rest of his life. At first he didn't want to talk about anything except testosterone. "I think it would help," he said expectantly. "I've read good things about what it can do and I'd like to give it a try."

I told him we weren't a testosterone clinic, but rather a health clinic, and that we would need to learn about the whole man so that we could work with him to come up with the right treatment for him. He was reluctant at first, but finally agreed to allow us to do our complete work-up.

We had Henry give us a full health history. We particularly looked for factors that might have caused early damage to his testes or caused them to function improperly. We asked about inflammations, undescended testes, and whether he had had mumps. We also asked if he had had a vasectomy or any other local traumas. Research has shown that these occurrences can cause problems later with healthy testosterone levels.

We then did a lifestyle and stress assessment study and talked with Henry about his depression and alcohol consumption and the stress he was feeling trying to keep up with a young wife.

Next we did a complete physical exam with special attention to his heart and arteries, testicles and penis. When we asked Henry to lie on his side on the examination table so we could do the digital rectal examination he seemed surprised. "I've had that done many times and I always had to pull down my pants and bend over the table," Henry told the doctor. "It was always uncomfortable and sometimes painful." We explained that we felt that being examined on the table, lying on his side, was generally a better method for most men. It is usually more comfortable and less painful, though some men say they prefer it the other way. After the exam Henry was amazed and delighted. "Hey, Doc, that wasn't bad at all," he said. "A heck of a lot more men would get examined if they knew they could do it like this. It really was painless and wasn't even very uncomfortable."

There were no abnormalities apparent from the digital exam, and we did a prostate specification antigen (PSA) blood test to confirm that there wasn't any sign of cancer.

Finally, we did a detailed fasting blood profile that included a hormone profile and full biochemistry panels to check on liver and kidney functions. We checked for blood fats and sugar, as well as hematological measurements of the red and white blood cells.

Everything looked fine, including the total testosterone level, but his bioavailable, or free, testosterone levels were low.

I told him that I wanted to learn more about his eating patterns, what he was doing for exercise, and his drinking habits, since they all had an effect on his overall health as well as what might be causing his symptoms. He seemed disappointed. "I know you'll probably want me to change my lifestyle, but couldn't I get started on the testosterone?"

Henry was like a lot of men who will deny for years that anything is changing in their lives or that they are having any problems, and when they finally do wake up, they want the quick fix with the least need for any real change. Fortunately for Henry, he was willing to explore other areas than just his hormones.

Over time he changed his eating habits dramatically, cutting down on his meat consumption and adding more fruits and vegetables. He began walking every day and started a program of workouts at the gym. We found that there was a good deal of hidden conflict in his relationship, which finally came out as we talked about how things were going sexually. Although the couple had enough money, both were rather bored with life. We helped them explore their interests, and Henry got involved in volunteer activities at the local high school.

We also began Henry on a regimen of testosterone replacement therapy (TRT). The total package of help seemed to do the trick. "I thought testosterone was all I needed," Henry told me after our six-month checkup. "But it was clear that there were other things that helped a lot. Changing my hormone levels seemed like a way to get things going fast, but it's clear to me now that exercise, diet, counseling, and finding new interests and direction for my life were equally important. I feel like a new man."

Although testosterone replacement therapy is not the only answer for those of us who want to stay vigorous and healthy as we age, it can be an important piece of the puzzle. For too long we have thought of hormone replacement therapy as something that only women need consider. We know now that hormones are also an important part of a man's life.

Testosterone treatments are now, and will become, an increasingly significant part of a wellness program for many men as we age. It is important, therefore, that we learn more about this hormone, which has gotten so much good and bad publicity over the years.

The 2,000-Year Search for the Essence of Manhood: The Testosterone Story

Two thousand years ago, the Greek scholar Pliny the Elder recommended eating animal testicles in order to promote sexual drive and interest. This practice is still popular in many countries—including Spain, where cooked bulls' testicles are served as the delicacy known as *cojones*. Not coincidentally, this is also a Spanish slang word for courage. Unfortunately, although testosterone is produced in the testes, it is quickly sent throughout the body in the bloodstream and little is in the organ at any one time.

A German chemist, Professor Adolf Butenandt, believed there must be a better way than scrounging up bulls' testicles, and kept working until he found it. He was able to devise a much easier and commercially more viable way of getting testosterone. It is essentially the same process that is used today.

Butenandt worked out the chemical structure of testosterone. He then produced it, as does the body, from cholesterol, its natural precursor. He sent his paper on the process and the structure to a noted German science journal on August 24, 1935.

Just one week later, a Swiss chemical journal received a paper from Leopold Ruzicka, a Yugoslavian chemist working for the Ciba pharmaceutical company in Zurich, announcing a patent on the method of production of testosterone from cholesterol. For this work, he and Butenandt received the Nobel Prize in 1939.

The scientific world (or at least the male majority) were overjoyed with these discoveries about testosterone. Various types of preparations and methods of administration were devised and thousands of men reported having improved health. Research on testosterone has had its ups and downs over the years, but now seems to be coming into its own.

"We think of testosterone as being the hormone of sexuality, but it is much more," says John E. Morley, M.D., professor of gerontology and director of the Division of Geriatric Medicine at St. Louis University and an expert in treating testosterone deficiency.

Morley says that as a junior tennis player back in the 1960s, he was able to beat the number one women's player in the world, Brazil's Maria Bueno. "It's not just a man's bulk that makes the difference in sports," he says. "It's his coordinated bulk. It's the thought processes that keep the body organized and in control. That's very visual-spacial, and it's very testosterone dependent." Morley believes that it is this aspect of testosterone's action that allows men to outperform women even in sports that don't rely solely on strength.

Another researcher, James Dabbs of Georgia State University, describes the unexpected serenity he noticed in men with high testosterone levels. When in competitive situations or under pressure, these men didn't get shaken and seemed to thrive. Think of St. Louis Rams quarterback Kurt Warner or Joe Montana, in his heyday for San

Francisco 49ers, calmly eluding tacklers in throwing the game-winning touchdown with seconds left in the contest. Picture Michael Jordan, with three men all over him, finding a crease in the defense, switching the ball from his right hand to his left, and putting in the winning shot. "Testosterone insulates these guys from distractions," says Dabbs.

Testosterone and Andropause

After my doctor prescribed testosterone for me, I noticed improvements in a number of areas of my life. My sexual interest and stamina increased, much to the delight of myself and my wife. I worried that the price I might have to pay was increased restlessness or irritability. Instead I found that I was more relaxed and serene, yet at the same time I had more energy and more excitement about life.

Although treatments for andropause have gotten much more attention in recent years in Europe it is still not accepted in the United States. Yet one of the first major studies on andropause—or the male climacteric, as it was called, appeared in the prestigious *Journal of the American Medical Association* in 1944. Titled "The Male Climacteric: Its Symptomology, Diagnosis and Treatment," it was written by two well-known American doctors, Carl G. Heller and Gordon B. Myers.

The symptoms that the authors attributed to the male climacteric were the same ones I described in chapter 3: fatigue, and impaired memory and concentration, nervousness, depression, hot flushes, and loss of libido and potency. Further, there was a significant improvement in symptoms when the men were given injections of testosterone. "Definite improvement in the symptomatology was noted by the end of the second week in all of the twenty cases treated," Heller and Myers reported. They also found that testosterone helped restore potency as well as libido.

Although doctors in the United States did not follow up on the initial work of Heller and Myers, testosterone replacement therapy did not die out.

Beginning in the 1950s a Danish doctor, Jens Møller, began treating older men with testosterone. Not only did it help with emotional and sexual problems, it also helped with severe circulatory problems. Though often in conflict with the conservative medical establishment in Denmark, he treated patients until his death in 1989. Dr. Møller's work is being continued by Dr. Michael Hansen.

It was Dr. Møller who first interested Dr. Malcolm Carruthers in doing studies on testosterone treatment in England. "From 1977 onwards I made many visits to his clinic in Copenhagen and saw for myself the dramatic benefits of testosterone treatment to the circulation," Dr. Carruthers recalls. "I came to realize how testosterone had its effects and helped Dr. Møller to edit the books he was writing."

At present Dr. Carruthers is one of the world's leading experts on treating aging men with testosterone. Unlike many of the antiaging gurus, Dr. Carruthers doesn't think hormones are the answer to everything: "Testosterone Replacement Therapy is but one of a broad range of methods for preventing and treating the andropause. Often, however, it proves the key to the door to recovery and puts men in a more positive frame of mind to undertake the other necessary steps, such as managing stress, drinking less, losing weight and exercising."

Treating Andropause with Testosterone

Since Dr. Carruthers's work in England has been well documented and his findings are easily verifiable, I would like to tell you more about the man and his work. I had corresponded with Dr. Carruthers for many years before I met him in Geneva at the World Congress on the Aging Male. Gray-haired, distinguished-looking, and outgoing, he seemed like a poster boy for the health benefits of using testosterone to age well. But his scientific background is also distinguished.

A prize-winning anatomist at medical school, he found few of the answers in studying the structure of man alone. After several years' clinical work in hospitals, general practice, and training as a specialist in chemical pathology, he became interested in the effects of stress in causing heart disease and other mind-made disorders. He became known as an international authority in this field, lectured in many countries around the world, and published over 100 scientific papers, presenting his ideas in several books.

He is now a consultant andrologist, a specialist in men's health, in his own clinic in London's Harley Street. He is finding further evidence proving the reality of male andropause, and he is developing new ways of restoring vitality and virility to men experiencing these problems.

He completed a study of 2,000 men going through andropause and presented his findings in his book *Maximising Manhood: Beating the Male Menopause.* His research findings need to be understood by men and women going through this change of life, as well as members of the medical profession who must become partners in treating them.

Dr. Carruthers reports that he has found all the men in his study to have improved after taking testosterone: "Andropausal symptom scores all fell statistically significantly and total sexual activity, which includes both intercourse and masturbation, increased."

It isn't surprising that physicians are beginning to offer testosterone for men as they have for women. "Testosterone decline is at the core of male menopause (and a key element in female menopause as well)," says Eugene R. Shippen, M.D., co-author of *The Testosterone Syndrome.* "Testosterone therapy has every prospect of becoming for men what estrogen therapy is now for millions of women."

"Testosterone supplementation for normal, healthy older men might some day rival that of estrogen for women," says Adrian Dobs, M.D., associate professor of medicine and director of the Endocrinology and Metabolism Clinical Trials Unit at Johns Hopkins.

"Various studies on men with low testosterone levels have confirmed that testosterone replacement restores sex drive, erection, orgasm, ejaculation, and nocturnal erections," Dr. Theresa Crenshaw reports. "The biggest effect is on sexual desire, as expressed by sexual thoughts and fantasies. Interestingly, studies also report a general improvement in mood."

Aubrey Hill, M.D., author of *The Testosterone Solution,* asks, "Is testosterone a 'fountain of youth'?" He answers his own question: "For many men, the answer is an emphatic yes. Testosterone replacement treatment can restore a man's testosterone level, and with it his sexuality and sense of masculinity, to that of a much younger man."

"Sexual dysfunction as well as virtually all the other symptoms of male menopause can be traced, at least in part, to an age-related decline in testosterone," say Jonathan V. Wright, M.D., and Lane Lenard, Ph.D., authors of *Maximize Your Vitality and Potency.* "One of the brightest lights in the treatment of male menopause today is the use of testosterone replacement therapy."

"Low testosterone is associated with decreased libido and erectile dysfunction," says Dr. John Morley. "Low testosterone with aging is also responsible for a decline in cognition, strength, and bone density. Replacing testosterone can help reverse these symptoms." Morley also notes that "testosterone replacement may have positive effects on cardiovascular disease in older males."

Is Testosterone Therapy Safe?

There is great concern among researchers, clinicians, and men (as well as women) who may consider taking testosterone about safety concerns. Dr. Carruthers, who has probably treated more men than any other doctor in the world, believes that testosterone is safe *when properly administered and under the direction of a physician trained in this area of medicine.*

This is a key point. As I said, too many people think that if hormones are natural they must be safe and therefore professional supervision is unnecessary. I'm continually asked by men who know I specialize in treating men with testosterone if they can get it over the counter. I tell them, unlike DHEA and melatonin, testostosterone cannot be obtained without a doctor's prescription. But even if it could, why would you want to take a powerful hormone without supervision from a professional who knows about the benefits *as well as* the drawbacks?

In treating thousands of men, Dr. Carruthers concluded: "Unpleasant side-effects were minimal, and limited to mild gastric irritation in a few patients. . . . On the safety side, blood pressures were unchanged or even fell slightly in the treatment group after six months," Dr. Carruthers concluded. "There were no adverse changes in blood fat patterns, glucose, liver function tests or any part of the detailed blood profile."

Doesn't Testosterone Cause Prostate Enlargement or Even Cancer?

Though there are concerns from some doctors that testosterone may cause an increase in prostate cancer, this did not seem to be the case in Dr. Carruthers's findings and those by many other physicians worldwide. Though it has been shown that testosterone will cause an existing cancer to grow more rapidly, there does not seem to be evidence to support the concern that testosterone will cause a cancer. "The early warning sign for prostate cancer, the prostate specific antigen [PSA], did not change at repeated tests up to five years," Dr. Carruthers found. "There were no signs of enlargement of the prostate clinically or on ultrasound scanning and no tumors developed."

In addition to his own studies, Dr. Carruthers has drawn on worldwide research to conclude that testosterone is safe. "Testosterone treatment has been used in a multitude of studies right round the world, often in much higher doses then those used to treat the andropause without any convincing evidence of it causing either benign enlargement or cancer as established from a literature search," says Dr. Carruthers.

Studies carried out in Amsterdam with one oral preparation of testosterone, Andriol, have not shown any adverse effects in serial tests in patients treated for over 20 years. The WHO multicenter trials of testosterone given in high doses to fit young men for a year or two have not shown any problems. Dr. Jens Møller, the Danish physician I mentioned earlier, gave very high doses of testosterone to over 3,000 men with circulatory disease over a 30-year period without prostate problems developing.

Research on testosterone replacement therapy continues around the world. Most researchers believe this treatment has great potential for good, but all want to be sure that we know as much as we can about potential risks. At present, the major researchers I have met believe that testosterone replacement therapy, along with other lifestyle supports, is helpful to many men as they age.

For Men Considering Testosterone Replacement Therapy: What You Need to Know

1. Do you have symptoms indicating possible testosterone deficiency?

I noted some of the main symptoms of andropause in chapter 3. Some of those signs overlap with the signs of testosterone deficiency. Here is a clinical questionnaire developed by Dr. Carruthers used to determine symptoms related to testosterone deficiency.

	None	Slight	Medium	Severe	Extreme
1. Fatigue, tiredness, loss of energy	____	____	____	____	____
2. Depression, low or negative mood	____	____	____	____	____
3. Irritability, anger, or bad temper	____	____	____	____	____
4. Anxiety or nervousness	____	____	____	____	____
5. Loss of memory or concentration	____	____	____	____	____
6. Relationship problems with partner	____	____	____	____	____
7. Loss of sex drive or libido	____	____	____	____	____
8. Erection or potency problems	____	____	____	____	____
9. Dry skin on face or hands	____	____	____	____	____

	None	Slight	Medium	Severe	Extreme
10. Excessive sweating day or night	_____	_____	_____	_____	_____
11. Backache, joint pains or stiffness	_____	_____	_____	_____	_____
12. Heavy drinking, past or present	_____	_____	_____	_____	_____
13. Loss of fitness	_____	_____	_____	_____	_____
14. Feeling overstressed	_____	_____	_____	_____	_____
15. The age you feel	30s	40s	50s	60s	70s
Total checks	_____	_____	_____	_____	_____
Multiply checks in each column by	0	1	2	3	4

If there have been adult mumps, orchitis or other testicular problems, a prostate operation or inflammation, persistent urinary infection, or vasectomy, each adds four points to the total scores.
Total score _____
Testosterone deficiency rating: 0–9 unlikely, 10–19 possible, 20–29 probable, 30–39 definite, 40+ advanced.

There is more information about interpreting the results of Dr. Carruthers's questionnaire on his web site. You can get the address by looking up the E-Medicine Andro Screen Center in the resource section at the end of the book.

2. Is your free or bioavailable testosterone level low?

It would be nice if there was a simple way to measure low testosterone levels. For years many doctors have gotten lab results that showed total testosterone was within normal limits and concluded that symptoms could not be the result of low testosterone. Now we know that we need more sensitive measures.

One of the main reasons that andropause has often gone undiagnosed is that unlike female menopause, where there is a clear and easily measurable precipitous drop in estrogen levels, it is difficult to show a similar drop in men who may have all the symptoms of testosterone deficiency.

To understand why a more sophisticated measure is needed, we need to delve a bit more deeply into the mechanisms of testosterone effects in the male body. The small but vital amounts of testosterone produced in the testes is quickly swept away in the bloodstream and carried to all parts of the body. That's why early attempts to get measurable quantities of testosterone by harvesting the testicles of animals yielded such meager results.

Most of the testosterone that circulates in the bloodstream is bound to a special carrier protein called sex hormone binding globulin (SHBG). The more SHBG there is, the less free, active, bioavailable testosterone is able to get out of the blood into the cells to do its job.

As we age, testosterone drops and SHBG increases. Although total testosterone may drop only slightly up to age 70, free testosterone drops more rapidly. In Dr. Carruthers's study he found that only 13 percent of the men showing symptoms of andropause had abnormally low levels of total testosterone, but 75 percent showed low levels of free testosterone.

It's crucial for men to know if their free testosterone level is low. This can be measured directly by some labs. It can also be gotten by taking the total testosterone and dividing by the SHBG level and multiplying by 100. Dr. Carruthers calls this the "free androgen index." "It is usually between 70 and 100 percent," says Dr. Carruthers. "It is when the free androgen index falls below 50 percent that symptoms usually appear."

To complicate the picture even more, there is a wide variation of normal testosterone levels between different men. We recommend that men have their free testosterone levels checked on a regular basis beginning at age 40 or earlier if symptoms are present. If symptoms develop, we can then look at how their testosterone levels have changed over time, not just a single reading.

3. Are there other possible causes for your symptoms?

As I have said, andropause is not just the result of hormonal changes. There are physical, dietary, psychological, interpersonal, social, and spiritual aspects. We explore all these areas before deciding where it is most appropriate to intervene.

For instance, a number of the symptoms associated with low testosterone, such as loss of libido, decrease in energy, or worry and anxiety, are also indicators of a period of spiritual questioning. This is a time to examine our lives, to come to peace with the past and to ask ourselves what we have yet to do in the future. It is a time where we are moving away from reliance on our physicality and learning more about our spirituality.

At our clinic all men are given a complete medical work-up, including a full health history. We check on other diseases a person may have, including heart disease and diabetes, as well as medications that a man may be taking. We know, for instance, that many diseases, as well as the medications to treat them, can contribute to erectile dysfunctions.

We do a complete examination for possible depression. Depression as well as the medications to treat it, are also implicated in erectile dysfunction.

We do a complete prostate examination, including blood tests to measure prostate specific antigen and a digital rectal examination of the prostate to rule out serious prostate enlargement or prostate cancer. Finally, we do a lifestyle and stress assessment test.

Even if a man has low testosterone it may be less intrusive, less expensive, and more effective to deal with other causes of his symptoms first. For instance, we often see men who come to the clinic with many of the symptoms listed above. After a complete evaluation we might find that the man was suffering from depression. It might make more sense to get him stabilized on an antidepressant before giving him testosterone.

We also talk with a man about issues of purpose and meaning. We want to acknowledge that he is not just a physical being, but also a spiritual being. We explore the ways in which the physical, emotional, and spiritual aspects of life are related.

4. Are there reasons you should not use testosterone?

It may be determined that your symptoms are being caused by testosterone deficiency, but it may not be wise to prescribe testosterone. Some men have low testosterone as a result of problems in the hypothalamus or pituitary glands. If this is the case, these brain problems should be treated first. If a man has a mild case of enlarged prostate, testosterone can still be prescribed. But if there are advanced obstructive symptoms, it should not.

If there is any indication of possible prostate cancer, testosterone should not be prescribed. Nor should it be prescribed for men who have breast cancer. If a man has sleep apnea, this condition should be treated before testosterone therapy is considered.

5. How should you decide if testosterone replacement therapy is right for you?

Ultimately each man must decide for himself after weighing the benefits and risks and talking things over with a competent doctor trained in this area of health care. No one should take testosterone or any other medication or supplement without consulting a professional trained in the field. Don't assume that if it's available, it must be safe. Don't assume if it's safe for someone else, it will be safe for you. Nor should you simply rely on the professional to give you what they think you need. This is your body and your life. You need to find health professionals who will work together with you.

6. If testosterone is recommended, what type should you use?

Testosterone can be given in the form of injections, pills, pellets, and through the skin in the form of patches, creams, and gels. Different preparations have different advantages and drawbacks. Shots, for instance, can last a week or two, but may be painful and give a high dose at first, then a drop at the end. Patches give a sustained dose, but may irritate the skin. The new gel, which has recently been released by Unimed Pharmaceuticals, goes right into the skin, but needs to be taken each day.

There is also disagreement about the benefits of using "natural" testosterone versus a synthetic preparation. (This same controversy is present in the use of female hormone replacement therapies.) Contrary to what some people are told, testosterone does not come from Spanish bulls' testicles extracted at the height of the mating season. All testosterone now used everywhere in the world is made from cholesterol, the same raw material the body uses to produce it.

Natural testosterone is made to be the exact chemical structure as testosterone in the body. The synthetic testosterones, also known as testosterone esters (testosterone enanthate, testosterone propionate, and testosterone cypionate), are modified to make them more active or longer-lasting. Since natural testosterone cannot be patented, changing the structures also allows pharmaceutical companies to patent the new product.

"For restoring sexuality and the diverse aspects of men's health known to deteriorate with age," says Dr. Jonathan Wright "natural testosterone, (and other natural androgens), as well as specific vitamins, amino acids, and herbal and botanical products are demonstrably more effective and safer in the human body than any synthetic 'hormones' and pharmaceutical drugs."

7. Once a therapeutic program has been decided upon, how often should you follow-up?

After three months, there should be an assessment to check the therapeutic response to the program. A complete prostate exam should be repeated, and if there are any abnormal signs testosterone should be discontinued.

After nine months, therapeutic response and prostate exams should be repeated and blood work should be done again.

If all indications are positive, you should come back every six months for evaluations to be sure no problems arise and to add more supports to the program as needed. You need to understand that taking testosterone is a long-term commitment. Once you begin you may need to continue for the rest of your life to keep receiving the positive effects.

Testosterone Replacement Therapy Pros

For men with a known testosterone deficiency, TRT may

- Improve energy and strength
- Increase bone density
- Enhance lean body mass
- Decease body fat
- Improve energy and mood
- Protect the heart
- Revive interest in sex
- Fight depression

Testosterone Replacement Therapy Cons

- Condition and treatment are not fully understood
- Most general practitioners are not familiar with use
- Data on long-term effects is sparse and not widely available
- Treatment may lower good (HDL) and bad (LDL) cholesterol, so patients with heart disease should be monitored closely
- Can increase fluid retention
- Can increase tumor growth in patients with breast or prostate cancer

What We Still Need to Learn

Good research of testosterone replacement therapy is still being conducted and results are still coming in. We are about where research on women and hormone replacement was 30 years ago. "We're a lot further along than we were five years ago when we weren't even sure if testosterone levels decreased with age," says Lisa Tennover, M.D., one of the world's foremost researchers on TRT. "However, we need a lot more data before we really understand the benefits and risks of testosterone replacement therapy.

While short-term data are encouraging and the few long-term experiences of clinicians have produced positive results, we still need large-scale, multicenter clinical trials to give us the data we need. With worldwide interest in men and aging and with a number of large pharmaceutical companies moving into the field, these kinds of trials are likely to occur in the near future. However, results take time to come in. What is a man to do in the meantime?

What Men Can Do Now

- Know your testosterone level. The sooner you check it out, the sooner you can establish your healthy baseline level.
- Maintain a healthy lifestyle. Testosterone replacement therapy is not a magic cure for years of unhealthy living.
- If you suspect you have low testosterone levels, check it out with your doctor. You may have to educate your doctor or find a specialist, such as an endocrinologist, who can work with you.

Whether you decide to take testosterone or any other hormones, staying physically fit will serve you well. There is increasing evidence that staying physically active and keeping your weight within normal limits can actually help keep your testosterone levels from falling so rapidly as you age.

CHAPTER 9

Health Is Not for the Weak—Let's Get Physical

Our power does not lie in our ability to remake the world, but rather in our ability to remake ourselves.

—Gandhi

KEN GOLDBERG is a man with a mission. He's a healthy, good-looking man who has been working with men most of his professional life. We met at the First National Conference on Men's Health. "I am a urologist who specializes in male health problems," he says. "The fact that men neglect their bodies is blatantly obvious to me every day. I was trained to correct those problems, but fixing the same ones over and over eventually became frustrating. I was like the mechanic who tries to salvage the car after the engine is burned up. The damage is already done."

A man who cares can't look at the continuing damage men do to themselves without being moved to action. "If men knew as much about their bodies as they do about their cars, they'd be a lot better off," says Dr. Goldberg. "We need to get men to realize that they are going to die if they don't make some pretty serious changes in the way they run their lives." This recognition formed the seed of a dream for a center that would speak to the specific needs of men.

In 1989 Dr. Goldberg opened the Male Health Center in Dallas, the first center in the country specializing in treating male health problems.

The purpose of the center is to help men live healthy and active lives. The center's strategies for improving men's health include early diagnosis and treatment of health problems, support during and after care, and education for men about their bodies so that future health problems can be avoided.

Unlike many medical approaches to health, Dr. Goldberg's program has a strong emphasis on physical exercise. In his characteristic straightforward approach to offering sound medical advice to men who have been trained to ignore their health, he offers the following suggestions:

> "Don't worry, I'm not going to tell you to exercise to save yourself from a heart attack. You already know that fit people may have half as many heart attacks and strokes. Right?
>
> Instead, I'm going to offer you some less-well-known but equally good reasons to put fitness on your daily to-do list:
>
> 1. Physical activity reduces your risk of colon cancer. According to a recent study in the journal *Cancer,* active men have much lower risk, even if they're overweight.
> 2. Exercise protects against, and may even reverse, diabetes. In a study of 22,000 doctors, those who exercised regularly had 42 percent fewer cases of diabetes.
> 3. Working out protects you from job burnout. Researchers at Tel Aviv University have found that active men are about half as likely to buckle under job stress.
> 4. Strength training may delay aging. When a group of 90-year-old men were put on a program of weight lifting, they increased strength by an average of 174 percent.
> 5. Fitness helps prevent you from getting sick. A study of 8,301 employees found that unfit people were 2.5 times as likely to call in sick.
> 6. Men who exercise are less likely to get prostate cancer. Among 20,785 Harvard alumni, only one man who burned up more than 4,000 calories a week exercising got prostate cancer. Those who burned fewer than 1,000 had 38 cases.
> 7. Exercise builds strong bones. Among 101 men 60 and older who took up exercise, bone density increased 19 percent on average.
> 8. Exercisers are depression resistant. The *American Journal of Epidemiology* reports that people who don't exercise are at "significantly greater risk of depression."

9. Exercise helps you go to sleep. Duke University scientists report that men who exercise fall asleep in half the time that it takes men who don't.
10. Fit people have better sex lives. When 78 inactive men took up exercising three or four days a week, their frequency of intercourse increased significantly.

What's more, you don't need to become a marathon runner to enjoy most of these benefits. The American Heart Association—which for the first time in 20 years has just added a heart disease risk factor to its list: inactivity—says that walking, gardening, dancing, croquet, and shuffleboard are all activities that offer significant health benefits."

If You Don't Get More Exercise You're Going to Die Sooner

Robert is a 58-year-old man who sat across from me at our first session. He was jovial, animated, and florid.

I listened to Robert laugh about his lack of exercise: "I know I really should get some exercise, but I'm afraid it will ruin my figure." Robert broke into peals of laughter. After listening to him go on for awhile, I looked him in the eye and spoke from my heart: "Robert, do you know what's going to happen to you if you don't get more exercise in your life? You're going to die!"

Robert stopped laughing. He looked like he'd just had a glass of cold water thrown in his face. He quickly regained his composure. "What do you mean, I'm going to die?" He smiled somewhat sheepishly. "Be serious, doc." I reached out and grabbed him by the spare tire encircling his ample waste. "I've never been more serious in my life. Without exercise you're on your way to an early grave. I don't want to see that happen. I can't stop you if you want to kill yourself, but I'm not going to let you go without a fight."

It was clear I had gotten through to him. He was shaken and definitely awake. "What do you say?" I asked him seriously. "Do you want to work with me to save your life?" Robert nodded and we began a program that, over time, proved successful. Exercise wasn't the only part of the program, but it was a crucial beginning.

I remember my own experience nearly 30 years earlier. I sat in my doctor's office asking that my allergy medications be refilled. I had had allergies and asthma since I was a kid and had been taking medications on and off since I was eight or nine years old. For most doctors, the visit was routine. I asked for my medications, got a prescription, and was out of the office in five minutes.

This was a new doctor whom I hadn't seen before, and much to my surprise he wanted to talk with me after his examination and before giving me my drugs. "How old are you?" he wanted to know. I told him I was 28. "How much exercise do you get?" I chuckled much like Robert had and gave my canned speech, which I was sure a fellow professional would well understand: "I joined the YMCA a while back, but I haven't had a chance to use it much. Work keeps me pretty busy, and when I'm home there's my wife and young son to deal with. I do as much as I can."

He nodded and continued. "Are you under a good deal of stress at work?" Clearly I was with someone who was well aware of what I was up against. "I sure am," I told him, shaking my head. "Some days it's all I can do to keep from exploding."

I waited for the look of understanding to express itself and for sympathetic words to be spoken. I got neither. Instead he looked me in the eye and said, "Do you know what's going to happen to a man of your age, with the kind of stressful job you have, and your lack of serious exercise?" I shook my head from side to side. I still had a smile on my face.

"You're going to die," he told me seriously. I felt like I had been slapped, the smile instantly gone from my face. "Get in a regular exercise program, at least three times a week. Come see me in three months. If you're still having problems with allergies we'll see what else we can do."

"You're not going to give me any medication?" I asked timidly. "No," he said. "You need exercise a lot more than you need medications. Medications will treat the symptoms. Exercise will treat the core of the problem." He finally smiled as he got up and shook my hand. "Good luck," he told me. "I know you'll do the right thing."

I felt stunned as I walked out of his office. No doctor had ever talked to me like that before. I didn't know whether to be infuriated or grateful. Somewhere deep inside I knew he was absolutely right. That day I went to the Y and signed up for an exercise class that met on Mondays, Wednesdays, and Fridays. It meant taking off a half hour from work on those days. When I caught myself saying, "I can't do that," I remembered the doctor's warning.

I started exercising and jogging three times a week. At the beginning I had to make myself leave work. It made it easier that it was "on doctor's orders." The first weeks were painful. I wheezed around the track, stopping often to walk. After a month I began to feel better. At the end of three months I felt wonderful, for the first time in a long time. I called the doctor to thank him. "I don't think I need the medications," I told him. "Good" was his only reply.

I wondered what kind of a doctor stays in business by taking time to talk to his patients about their lives, refusing to give medications, prescribing exercise, and encouraging his patients *not* to come back for follow-up visits. One that believes in helping his patients live long and well, I guessed. Whatever his motivations, I was extremely grateful. So was my wife, who could look forward to many years with her partner. So was my little boy, who could look forward to many years with his father.

The "Magic Pill" That Will Keep You Healthy

We all would like to find that magic pill that we can take that will keep us healthy. It may be that exercise provides the magic. So, listen up guys: If there's one thing you can begin right away to improve your health, it's exercise. Not convinced yet? Read on.

Recent research findings validate the tremendous value of exercise. We don't have to be extreme athletes to get the benefits. Walking is free and easy and helps us to live long and well. If you have been exercising, keep it up. If you have been a couch potato, it's never too late to begin.

A major study of over 7,000 men in England tracked the exercise habits and health of these men for nearly 20 years. The study revealed a strong link between exercise and survival. Even light exercise was protective, reducing the risk of death by 39 percent; moderate exercise was even better, cutting the mortality rate by 50 percent. Even men who were sedentary when the study began and started exercising 12 to 14 years later enjoyed a 45 percent lower mortality rate than those who remained sedentary.

These kinds of findings have been validated in studies from the Netherlands, Norway, and the United States. The *Harvard Men's Health Watch,* which reported the findings in their April 2000 issue, concluded: "From both sides of the Atlantic, the message is clear. Exercise is beneficial for all stages of life, and it's never too late to start. Aerobic exercise is the best way to reduce the risk of cardiovascular disease and extend life expectancy. Although many forms of activity can fit the bill, walking will do just fine; 45 minutes a day is optimal. Add stretching for flexibility and light resistance training for strength, and you'll have a balanced program for your whole body."

I have a friend, Bill, who is very overweight. He has tried all kinds of methods to lose weight with little success. I suggested he begin regular exercise. He told me he was too heavy to exercise, that it wouldn't do him any good until he had lost weight. Recent research shows that Bill, and millions like him, are wrong.

In the February 5, 2001, issue of *Time* magazine there was a report on a 1999 study of 25,000 men whose average age was 44 years. "All other things being equal," the research demonstrated, "men who were obese and physically fit had about the same risk of death over a 10-year period as men who were both physically fit and of normal weight." The study also found another related fact: "Men of normal weight who were unfit were twice as likely to die as the obese but fit men."

If you are as surprised by these findings as I was, read the preceding paragraph again. What it says to me is that if we want to be healthy, exercise may be *the* key element in the program. "It's pretty clear that if you follow a healthy diet and don't smoke, but don't exercise, you are still at high risk of chronic illness," says Steve Blair, one of the authors of the study and the director of research at Cooper Institute in Dallas, Texas.

Why wait, start now. You'll be happy you did.

We Are Built to Be Physical

If you want to know how to keep a piece of machinery running, it is a good idea to know something about how it was designed to operate. It's even better if there is an owner's manual that goes with it to tell you how to keep it running well. Our human ancestors have been on the planet for nearly 4 million years. If we knew how we were meant to be, it would go a long way in helping us stay healthy.

Three modern-day scientists have tackled the problem: S. Boyd Eaton, M.D., a radiologist; Marjorie Shostak, an anthropologist; and Melvin Konner, M.D., Ph.D., one of the leading experts in the emerging field of evolutionary psychology. Together they wrote *The Paleolithic Prescription: A Program of Diet and Exercise and a Design for Living.*

"Our genetic constitution has been selected to operate within a milieu of vigorous, daily, and lifelong physical exertion," say Eaton, Shostak, and Konner. "The exercise boom is not just a fad; it is a return to 'natural' activity—the kind for which our bodies are engineered and which facilitates the proper function of our biochemistry and physiology."

Physical fitness has three main components: cardiorespiratory (aerobic) endurance, muscular strength, and flexibility.

Good cardiorespiratory endurance means that activities requiring stamina (such as soccer, swimming, running, racquetball, and basketball) can be maintained for relatively prolonged periods.

Muscular strength usually peaks between the ages of 20 and 30, and declines steadily thereafter. Yet regular exercise can reduce the rate of decline. Strong muscles guard against injuries and exercise helps keep our bones strong and protects us against osteoporosis. It also keeps us from getting that potbelly as we age. The more muscle we have, the more calories our bodies uses, *even when we're resting.* So preserving muscle keeps our body running, even when we're not.

Yet one of the most important aspects of our exercise program should be flexibility. Flexible bodies are limber, supple, and graceful. And, we might add, sexy at any age. One of the prime problems men have as we age is with our backs. This seems to be one of the side effects of having only recently, in evolutionary time, begun to walk upright.

Anyone who has ever had a back go out, and that seems to be almost all of us over 50, knows it's difficult to feel strong and manly, much less sexy, when it hurts to move. "There's definitely a strong connection between good back flexibility and great sex," says James White, Ph.D., professor emeritus at the University of California, San Diego. "A lover with a stiff back is an oxymoron."

Walter M. Bortz II is a 70-year-old who looks like a 50-year-old and has the physical strength and endurance of many 30-year-olds. He is also the author of *We Live too Short and Die too Long* and *Dare to Be 100.* He is a member of the teaching faculty at Stanford University Medical School and a practicing physician who says he learns most from his patients, the majority of whom are older than he is. "Fitness for a young person is an option," says Dr. Bortz. "Fitness for older people is an imperative."

His advice on exercise is down to earth and sensible. "If you are planning a long trip, you want to be sure that whatever kind of conveyance you are planning to use for your trip is sturdy enough to carry you the whole way and not leave you broken down before the trip is over," he tells us. "But what if your trip is 100 years long and your vehicle is your body? Will it last you your full lifespan?"

The most common reason men give for not exercising is "I don't have time." That's been my excuse. Come to think of it, I'm doing it right now. I've been sitting here for hours working on this book. My back is beginning to ache, and my neck and shoulders are stiff. I think I'll follow the doctor's orders right now. I'm going to save the file, turn my computer off, change into shorts, and go for a run. I better practice what I preach. How about you?

—∞—

ACTION OPTION

Overcome Your Obstacles to Exercise

Write down the reasons you give yourself for not exercising more. Then list the reason why more exercise would be good for you.

—∞—

Are You Ready to Get Physical?

I had known Rodney for many years. He was a very successful businessman who had worked for a large corporation for many years before starting his own company when he was 40 years old. There were a number of years of struggle, but by age 50, Rodney could say that his consulting company had "made it."

When he was working in corporate America and had long but regular business hours we often exercised together. We would play ball after work and would often run together on weekends. But once he started working for himself he was always "too busy."

Now he had time and seemed to want to develop his physical fitness, but he still couldn't get himself going. Although he still looked good for a man of his age, he complained that he was putting on weight. "It just seems to creep up a little each year," he would tell me. When we'd run or play ball, he'd quickly tire and often complain the next day that he was stiff and everything hurt. Sprained ankles, pulled groin muscles, and lower back injuries were common occurrences.

Does Rodney sound like anyone you know? Do you see any similarities to your own life? If so, I invite you to join Rodney as he develops his program for physical well-being. Think back to or reread the steps for successful change I outlined in chapter 1 and follow along with Rodney as he moves through each one. You might want to write out your own answers to the questions.

The 11 Steps to Physical Health

1. Feel discomfort about your physical health.

After helping people change their lives for over 35 years, I have found an important truth. No matter how unhealthy a person may be, physically, emotionally, and spiritually, until he or she *feels* uncomfortable with his or her condition nothing will ever change. Spouses, friends, family, and doctors can all tell you that you need to do something, but until you feel the pain of your present situation you will stay just the way you are.

"The truth is," Rodney told me, "until recently I was so wrapped up in my business I wasn't even aware that I was getting out of shape." Often the awareness that our present life is painful dawns on us in little bursts of awareness. It's like there is a break in the cloud cover and the sun shines its light on our lives. "The day after we'd run or play ball my body ached and I was so stiff I couldn't sit comfortably," Rodney recalled. "I'd be aware of my pain at those times, but I'd get an important phone call and get lost in the next big project."

Often this first stage can last for many months or even years. Unfortunately we are very good at cutting ourselves off from the awareness of our pain. Many of us wait until there is a major breakdown before we can really feel it. I had to wait until the doctor told me I was going to die if I didn't get more exercise. Rodney didn't wait that long. I hope you are as smart as Rodney.

2. Think about how you would like your physical health to be.

The day after one of our infrequent runs, Rodney and I were having lunch together. He was obviously stiff and in pain. Rather than talk about how much he hurt, which he often did at these times, I asked him to think about how he would like things to be. After looking a bit perplexed, Rodney began to mull it over. "I want to feel good," he began somewhat hesitantly, but then began to warm to the subject. "I want to be able to play hard without waking up the next day in pain. I want to feel more alive. I want to move like the athlete I once was."

As Rodney talked I began to see the excitement and fire that had made him such a successful businessman focused on his physical health. I liked what I was hearing. Too often we use our passion, courage, and commitment to get things done in the outside world while failing to apply those qualities to our own lives.

3. Get specific about what you'd like to change about your physical health.

I smiled at Rodney. His enthusiasm was infectious. I encouraged him to get specific about what he wanted to change.

"Well, I'd like to exercise more regularly," he began. "I know I'm always going to hurt afterward if I only get out there once a month or so.

"I want to be more flexible," he continued. "I want to be able to touch my toes when I bend over. I want to avoid injury, play without pain, and feel energized afterward. I don't want to feel stiff and tired the next day."

4. Prioritize your desires about physical health.

One of the things that often keeps us from being successful with a physical health program is that we try to do everything at once. We want to make up for lost time and get fit fast. We need to remind ourselves that we didn't get out of shape overnight and we won't get in shape overnight.

I asked Rodney about what was most important to him and where he might begin. "I guess if I had to start with one thing," he said, "I would want to be able to play racquetball regularly. It gives me a good workout. I like being with other guys and I like the competition." Rodney offered this last statement with a little half smile that I was familiar with.

Although Rodney and I are not nearly as competitive as we once were, we still like to feel the excitement of going up against an opponent. Now we compete for the fun of the game, not to see who could dominate his opponent.

5. Pick a desire you have for physical health and examine the benefits and drawbacks of taking action.

As is true of most of us, by the time we got to this step Rodney wanted to go past this one and get right to work. We're action oriented. Once we get rolling we want to start immediately. I explained the importance of this step. This is the one that will keep you going when you feel like quitting, and believe me there will be times when you won't want to do the things you know are good for you.

So let's look at the benefits Rodney believed he would receive from playing racquetball regularly:

- I will get away from the stresses of work.
- I will have fun with guys I like.
- I'll be in the gym so I can do other things like swim, sit in a hot tub, get a massage, and lift weights.
- My body will feel more flexible.
- I'll probably feel less stressed at work.
- It might encourage my wife to get more exercise herself.
- I'll be a good role model for my children.

- I'll be healthier in other areas of my life.
- I might lose some weight.

After completing his list of benefits, Rodney was really champing at the bit. Once again I had to restrain him. I told him, "If exercise were nothing but benefits you'd be doing it already, and you'd do it your whole life. But there are some drawbacks as well. Think about what those might be." This was a more difficult list to make than the first one. Rodney needed some help in getting it done, but once he got the idea, the perceived drawbacks began to become evident, and he came up with this list:

- Although it is stressful, I really do love my work. There are times I just lose myself in a project and don't want to do anything else.
- I like people, but I do so much people work on my job I often just want to be alone.
- I'm afraid I wouldn't just focus on racquetball. Since I'm already at the gym I'd pressure myself to do "everything," then I'd feel overwhelmed and stop coming altogether.
- My wife already complains that I'm not spending enough time with her; if I took more time to go to the gym, it might make her even more unhappy.

(Sometimes the perceived drawbacks are hidden from consciousness and need supportive probing to get at. When Rodney talked about his wife, Barbara, there seemed to be some tension that was just below the surface. When I asked how things were going he said everything was fine, but when I probed a bit more deeply, he acknowledged that it seemed they had grown somewhat distant over the last few years. This discussion led to some other perceived drawbacks to improving his physical health that Rodney was not aware of at first.)

- If I'm fit and trim and Barbara is not, it may increase tension and distance between us.
- Barbara has always been somewhat jealous. There are always a number of nice-looking ladies at the gym. Going more often might increase Barbara's jealousy.

(This last drawback came very reluctantly. Sometimes it's the less-conscious, deeper concerns that are at the root of our resistance to changing our health patterns for the better.)

- It's not just Barbara's jealousy I'm worried about. I find myself more and more attracted to other women. I love my wife, and I don't want to put pressure on our marriage. I guess I'm worried that if I spent more time at the gym I might be tempted more to look and if I looked . . .

(What can begin as a simple process of looking at the pros and cons of playing racquetball can open up other aspects of our lives. Remember I told you all the levels of health are related? Here's another example. After we completed this part of the exercise, Rodney agreed that he and Barbara needed to have a real heart-to-heart talk about the state of their marriage.

There was a break of almost six weeks before Rodney came back to complete the process. He told me he was glad now that he had stayed with the steps. He and Barbara had talked, taken a week off to be alone and reevaluate their marriage, and come back closer than they had ever been. Rodney was now ready for the next six steps.)

6. Make the decision to improve your physical health.

Most of us make our decision to change without honestly looking at the benefits and drawbacks. As with Rodney, it is usually the *unacknowledged* drawbacks that get in the way of our being successful. Now that you've really looked at the two lists, the benefits and the drawbacks to a program of physical health, what do *you* really want to do? All of life has its trade-offs. No one can really know what someone else's internal balance sheet is like. Sometimes we don't even know ourselves.

However, when we really get a complete look at the benefits versus the drawbacks of changing our lives, we are in a position to make an honest decision. I asked Rodney to consider his lists—not just the number of responses on each side of the ledger, but how important each one is. There may be 10 reasons to make a change and only a single reason not to. But if that one reason is a big one, it may outweigh the other 10.

"Well, I can see now that making the change I wanted wasn't the obvious slam dunk I had assumed it to be," Rodney said slowly. "But, yes, I still want to make the change." I could see that Rodney's hesitation was because he was really considering his choices. When he said yes, I could tell he was serious. He was going into the game with his eyes wide open and therefore was likely to succeed.

7. Decide on a goal for physical health.

Before deciding on a goal for Rodney's physical health, we needed to talk about some other related issues. We talked about his need for regular activity. We talked about his job schedule. We talked about his need to spend time with Barbara. We talked about the possible distractions of being around young, attractive women.

I told Rodney that it wasn't enough to say he wanted to get away from the stresses of work, or to have more fun time with the guys, or to get his body feeling more flexible. He needed a specific goal.

After discussing all the issues involved, Rodney decided that his goal was to play racquetball three times a week.

8. Develop an action plan for physical health.

I told Rodney that playing three times a week was a worthy long-term goal, but he needed a specific action plan that would take him one step at a time to achieving that goal. Many of us want to have it all now. We don't want to take things step-by-step.

I explained to Rodney that to play racquetball three times a week, to enjoy it while he played, and to feel good afterward, he would need to have three parts to his exercise program.

The first was to improve his flexibility. The second was to become stronger. The third was to work up to his goal a little at a time.

We came up with the following action plan:

- For the first week Rodney would come to the gym once. He would do a series of yoga postures for 20 minutes that would increase his flexibility, making it less likely that he would feel stiff, sore, or get injured.
- For the second week Rodney would come twice. On one day he would do the yoga exercises. On the second day he would work with weights. This would both improve flexibility and strength.
- During the third week Rodney would come three times. On one day he would do yoga. On the next day he would lift weights. On the third day he would lift weights, do yoga, and play racquetball.
- During subsequent weeks Rodney would add time in each of the three activities so that there was a good balance.

I emphasized the importance of stretching before and after playing ball. Most sports injuries occur because we don't warm up before and cool down afterward. This is not just a matter of getting our bodies ready to play, but also involves our getting ourselves mentally prepared. When we rush right from the office to the gym, our minds are as stiff as our bodies. We need to loosen both up if we are going to stay fit.

9. Anticipate obstacles and come up with answers to staying with the physical health program.

One of the major benefits of examining both the pros *and* cons of our physical health program is that we can see where we might run into trouble and plan a strategy in advance. Here is what Rodney came up with:

Obstacle: I get caught up with projects at work.
Answer: Put my gym schedule on my work calendar so that I don't book activities during those times.
Obstacle: I need more time alone.
Answer: Take a half-hour walk alone after I leave the gym before returning to work.
Obstacle: I would do too much while I was at the gym.
Answer: Keep a card with my activity schedule on it. Do only those activities listed on my card for the first six months.
Obstacle: Barbara would feel I'm spending too much time away.
Answer: Invite her to come with me.
Obstacle: If I get healthier and Barbara doesn't, there will be more distance between us.
Answer: Quit nagging her about exercise. If I set an example rather than pushing on her, maybe she'll want to get fitter on her own.
Obstacle: Barbara gets jealous of other women.
Answer: Take her out on a date once a week, no matter how busy I am. Let her know how special she is and how much she means to me.
Obstacle: My own fears of my attractions to other women.
Answer: Be sure there are not unspoken barriers with Barbara. Keep our marriage strong.

10. Get supports to keep your health program going.

Many of us have the false belief that if we are really motivated to change we should be able to do it on our own. The truth is that most of the changes we need help with can benefit from ongoing support. Rodney said he got a lot of support from having someone take him through these 11 steps. He also recognized that keeping his program for physical health was important to do and important to maintain.

Here's what he decided would help keep him on track:

- Telling friends that he was committing to a program of physical health.
- Asking a few close friends to call him up regularly and ask about his progress.
- Keeping a log on how he felt each day before his workout and after it.
- Asking his wife to encourage his program. (After Rodney had talked with Barbara and they had cleared up some relationship blocks, it was very easy for her to give him the support he was asking for.)
- Monitoring his progress.

To keep a program moving forward, we need to monitor our progress. The benefit of such monitoring is that it allows us to see if we are beginning to get off track before we go too far afield. It also helps us to reward ourselves by noticing our positive changes. Rodney decided to check in with me every three months to get a boost of encouragement and to help him evaluate how he was doing.

11. Maintain a positive program throughout our lives.

How many times have we started a physical fitness program, or any kind of health program, only to find that it fizzled out after a few months? The key to maintaining a program throughout our lives is to begin to build it into how we live. I've been running regularly now for over 30 years.

At first it was a program to keep me fit. To help make it a part of my life, I signed up for a class that met three times a week and included exercise and light jogging. I liked the contact with other men and being able to get outside and destress after a hard day at the office.

Having a regular class to attend helped keep me motivated after my program had been completed. Later I was given the opportunity to help teach the class. This gave me even more incentive to show up regularly and to stay in good shape as an example to the others who attended the class.

Regular exercise is now as much a part of my life as brushing my teeth every day. I don't have to try to do it, and I don't worry that I'll lose my motivation. Rodney decided to get a two-year membership to the health club. "I know if I pay my money up front, I'll be more motivated to keep things going," he said.

Dealing with Chronic Pain: One of the Primary Obstacles to Staying Physically Fit

One in five of us suffers from chronic pain that can last for weeks, months, and even years and can limit our ability to do even simple physical tasks. One in four of us who are over 65 suffer. One in four of us take some kind of medication on a daily basis to deal with pain. It's difficult to develop and maintain a program of physical fitness if it hurts when we move.

Most of us grew up learning to ignore pain. We played through pain and even saw pain as a marker of progress. "No pain, no gain" was our motto. We laughed and ridiculed our buddies if they complained about being hurt, and would suffer in silence to keep from being the focus of their ridicule.

As young men it seemed that there were few consequences to our attitude. We got injured, we would grin and bear it, we would recover, and we would look forward to the rough-and-tumble of the next time. Most all our pain was acute pain. This is pain caused by sprained ankles, scraped knees, and sore muscles.

But the chronic pain we associate with our aching backs, our swollen joints, and our bad knees is something different. Acute pain has biological value. It tells us to pay attention, seek help, and stop what we are doing. Chronic pain persists continuously or intermittently for months or years, long past the time when it might be biologically useful, and it doesn't go away with time or rest.

Until recently the medical profession, most of whose members are male, seemed to take a traditional male attitude toward pain. If the cause of pain was not obvious and related to a specific disease or injury, many doctors concluded that those suffering were "whiners" or "malingerers" or that the pain was "all in our head." Since that's what a lot of us guys believe already, we have tended to ignore chronic pain and suffer in silence.

New research shows that chronic pain is not just in our head but affects our entire body. Not only that, but chronic pain syndromes can actually change the way our body's pain-sensing mechanisms and our natural pain-relieving systems operate. The result is that the nervous system becomes more sensitive to pain and less receptive to the brain chemicals that moderate or turn off pain.

In other words, the more pain, the less gain. Chronic pain can feed on itself and actually change the structure of our nervous system so that the longer it lasts the more pain it produces. Chronic pain can actually cause nerves to sprout sensitive new endings. It can cause receptors for natural pain-relieving compounds to deaden. As pain becomes chronic, it can be triggered by stimuli as benign as a cool breeze.

I remember having an experience like that when I had back spasms that lasted for months. It seemed like the littlest thing would set them off. I got so I almost didn't want to move at all for fear I would do something to trigger the pain. Since one of the joys of my life is running and playing ball at the gym, not being able to do these things increased my anxiety and depression, which in turn made me even more fearful.

In this way chronic pain has some of the characteristics of cancer. If untreated, it takes over our whole system and causes increasing damage to our body, mind, and spirit. The old adage to "grin and bear it" when dealing with our pain is just as illogical and destructive as it would be if we applied it to dealing with cancer.

Anyone who has cancer should be treated, and anyone suffering chronic pain should likewise be treated. In fact, most pain experts treat chronic pain as a disease in its own right, not just a symptom of something else. At our clinic we use a holistic approach that includes addressing the physical and psychological aspects of pain, the emotional distress that is the result of living with chronic pain, and the social and cultural factors that influence our perceptions and response to pain.

ACTION OPTION

Talk about Chronic Pain

Talk to a friend or a loved one about the experience of chronic pain in your life. Discuss pain that you experience now. Share the things that you have tried that have helped, as well as the things you have tried that have not helped. If it has been some time since you have talked to a health care professional about your chronic pain, make an appointment to see someone.

Isn't There an Easier Way to Stay Physically Healthy?

There *is* an easier way. And you are already doing it. If you've survived this long in life, there are many things you are doing right. If you were a total physical wreck, you probably wouldn't be reading this book. Take a moment to think of the physical things that you already do. Even the most inactive of us do some walking. Most of us stretch from time to time. We even lift heavy objects once in awhile.

I'm not asking you to start from scratch. You're already doing some good things. I'm offering you an opportunity to expand and deepen what you are already doing. If you need a bit more incentive, listen to Rodney's final words on the subject: "I started this program because I wanted to feel better after a game. I got that and much more. This process has helped Barbara and me get closer together. We have regained the intimacy I thought we had lost." Rodney stopped and I saw that sly look I know well. "And I'm not exactly sure how it works, but our sex life has become quite wonderful."

PART IV

The Men Alive Program for Emotional and Spiritual Health

CHAPTER 10

Understanding Our Feelings and Recognizing Our Emotional Pain

> The tragedy of life is in what dies inside a man while he lives—the death of genuine feeling, the death of inspired response, the death of awareness that makes it possible to feel the pain or glory of other men in oneself.
>
> —Norman Cousins

Getting in Touch with Our Emotional Body

I've always prided myself on being the kind of man who got things done. I knew I could achieve anything I set my mind to and tasted success early. What I was not aware of was that stress went along with success. There was never enough time to get everything done. I was driven by deadlines but told myself I thrived on the pressure. It didn't occur to me that my stomach problems, sleepless nights, and periodic attacks of asthma had anything to do with the stress I was under.

Once our two children arrived, I felt even more driven. I vowed that I would not turn out like my father, unable to support his family. I worked overtime whenever we needed money—and we always seemed to need more. After awhile this way of life seemed normal. If someone would have told me I was under stress, I would have laughed. "Are you kidding?" I would have told them. "I feel great."

I knew I *had* to stay strong, keep going, make a living, support my family, be successful, show the world. Below the surface of my awareness was the need to prove to my mother that I would not disgrace the family by turning out like my father. Also buried deep was my desire to prove to my father that I could be a better man than he had been. And many, many layers down was the fear that if I ever slowed down I would end up just like him, locked up in a mental hospital.

If things had gone my way, I would have continued to strive for success, run from the stress, and keep my fears from my childhood buried. However, life events conspired to wake me up. Thank God they did.

The Wake-up Call

A number of years ago one of our sons was having trouble with drug use and went to a treatment program for help. As part of the program there were two weekends that were devoted to family involvement. My wife, Carlin, and I were eager to attend to learn more about what we could do to support his recovery. We were surprised to learn that part of the education we received was an opportunity to look at our own mental health issues.

We learned that many parents who have adult children with alcohol or drug problems often have problems of their own. Some involve drugs, but others have psychological issues often related to anxiety and depression. Each of the parents was given a questionnaire to fill out, which helped the staff see if there were indications of depression, a condition we learned was very prevalent throughout the population.

We found that Carlin scored high on the depression test, while my scores were low. I was surprised to find that my wife had indications of depression. She hadn't seemed depressed to me. I figured if she was unhappy she'd tell me. When Carlin spoke to one of the professional staff at the program, the woman told her that she suspected Carlin was depressed from having seen her interact over the two weekends we were present. I wondered how I had missed something that seemed so obvious to a stranger.

The *American Medical Association Encyclopedia of Medicine* defines depression as "feelings of sadness, hopelessness, pessimism, and a general loss of interest in life, combined with a sense of reduced emotional well-being." Like so many people who live busy lives, I hadn't taken time to be aware of what was going on inside my wife's psyche.

As we drove back home from the treatment center, Carlin shared with me the feelings that had built up over many years. I was amazed to see how much sadness she had been carrying and how much her mind was preoccupied with feelings of worry that she couldn't do anything right. Although I acted as sympathetic and protective as I could be, secretly I felt superior that I was able to handle my feelings without letting them get me down.

I kept thinking about her high score and my low score on the depression questionnaire. Though I knew the thought was irrational, somehow I felt that a lack of depression made me a superior person. I felt that in the game of life I had the better score, and it somehow indicated that I was a better human being.

As a mental health professional, I felt I had learned about depression and so had become inoculated against the disease. Never mind that depression was everywhere in my family, on both my mother's and father's sides. I saw myself as a healer who could work among people with a disease and never catch it himself. I was too busy. I was too dedicated to helping others. I was too pure at heart. I was too smart to let myself get caught by depression. Oh, was I ever wrong.

Depression: The Silent Killer of Men

Depressed people have often been told to "just cheer up." But we know now that isn't possible because depression is caused by a disruption in the chemistry of the brain. Only by restoring chemical balance can we truly hope to cure depression. We now know that there is a strong inborn component to depression and that the susceptibility to depression runs in families.

Yet most men who suffer from depression aren't even aware that they have it. They often don't recognize themselves when they hear the classic symptoms of major depression, such as persistent sad moods, recurrent thoughts of death, diminished ability to think or concentrate, feeling worthless, sleeping too much, low energy, loss of pleasure in life's activities, and significant weight loss or gain.

I believe too many men, particularly in the midlife years, are suffering and dying from unrecognized depression. Consider the following facts:

- Eighty percent of all suicides in the United States are men.
- The rate of suicide for men 45 to 64 is *three* times higher than the rate for women of the same age. For men over 65 the rate is nearly *seven* times higher.

- A large Swedish survey found a history of depression in men and women multiplied the risk for suicide *78-fold* compared to those with no such history.
- Mood disorders are the "common cold" of mind-body illnesses and more than 20 million Americans will suffer an episode of depression during their lifetimes.
- Since the turn of the century, each successive generation has doubled its susceptibility to depression.
- Sixty to 80 percent of people with depression never get help.
- For those who seek professional care, it may take up to 10 years and three doctors to make the correct diagnosis.
- Procrastination is a hallmark of depression. The depressive puts things off until they seem insurmountable. This reinforces his feelings of self-blame and despair.
- Men often think of depression as a "woman's ailment" and are reluctant to seek help even when they know they suffer from depression.
- Most men are not aware that they are depressed and so never have the opportunity to get help.
- Eighty to 90 percent of those seeking help can get relief from depression.

Healer, Heal Thyself

I was one of those men. Many years after my wife had sought and received help for her depression and after many years of her telling me she thought I was depressed, too, I was still insisting that "I'm not depressed, damn it, leave me alone." I clung to my score on the depression test I had taken years earlier as "proof" that I was OK. I was like a drowning man going down for the third time, insisting that "I'm OK. I'm fine. I'm just out for a swim. I can handle things. Really, I'm fine . . . glug, glug, glug."

I was irritable and angry all the time. But there were reasons for that. I had a lot of stress on my job, raising kids was not easy, and my wife was going through menopause and having her own problems. "Who wouldn't be angry?" I would bellow to anyone who would listen. Carlin received the brunt of the anger, which she fought to deflect. But what did she expect? She kept doing all these things that irritated me. If she'd just be nicer, more loving, more interested in sex, everything would be OK. (It never occurred to me that my constant anger made it nearly impossible for her to be nicer, more loving, more interested in sex.)

Yes, I was worried most of the time. But wasn't that normal? After all, I had to worry about making enough money to pay the bills. I had to worry about losing my job in an economy where someone else got rich while most of us got poorer and poorer. I worried about the children, grown and gone, but still needing help. I worried about my aging parents. I worried about the state of the world. I worried about getting old. I worried that I worried so much.

It never occurred to me that my worry was a symptom of an inner problem, not a response to problems that someone else was causing in my life. Two people helped turn my life around. One was Carlin, who never gave up trying to help me see that the problem wasn't her, or him, or my mother, or my job, or the world. The problem was in me. The other person was Buck, a client that Dr. Edward M. Hallowell describes in his book *Worry.*

Buck had gone to see Dr. Hallowell for help with his son's learning disabilities. I immediately felt a connection since I had a daughter with similar problems. Dr. Hallowell describes his meeting with Buck.

> It became clear right away that the man was more upset than he knew. He arrived for his appointment twenty minutes late, irritated at the traffic that had slowed him down, and he was angry at the fact that life was presenting him with yet another problem. He was sweating and out of breath just in telling me of his annoyances. . . . After about ten minutes I asked him how he was."
>
> "Me?" he replied in surprise. "How am I? Now that you ask, I'm a mess."
>
> "What's going on?" I asked.
>
> He took a deep breath and let it out though pursed lips. Then he took another breath and let that one out more easily. "I have so much going on," he said. "I don't know where to start. Just coming here to see you required major changes and compromises. I'm overextended. I don't know if I can make it. I can't think about it or I'll get overwhelmed. Let's talk about my son."
>
> "How are you sleeping?" I asked, ignoring his request.
>
> "Hardly at all," he replied. 'I stay up into the night worrying. It is driving me crazy. But why complain? What can I do but keep trying? I have no choice."

As I read about Buck, I thought, "That's me. He's talking about me." I also thought about my father. Those could have been his words just before he tried to kill himself. I shuddered, and something broke through my wall of denial.

"This man—Buck—had a choice but he didn't know it," wrote Dr. Hallowell. "He was depressed. He was running on empty and was about to run out. It is a fact that some highly responsible men and women such as Buck tend not to recognize depression in themselves because they are too busy to stop and consider their state." Now I felt Dr. Hallowell and Buck were speaking directly to me, and I was beginning to shed my tears as I began to shed my protective armor.

"They work harder and harder and cut themselves less and less slack," wrote Dr. Hallowell, "until some catastrophic event stops them dead—sometimes literally—in their tracks. They may have a heart attack or a stroke, they may get fired, their spouse may walk out, they may collapse in exhaustion, they may have an automobile accident, they may exercise disastrously poor judgment, or they may accidentally on purpose commit suicide. These are some of the potential, dire consequences of unrecognized depression."

By then I was weeping. "God, could I really be depressed and not know it?" I reluctantly went to Carlin and asked her for the name of the doctor she had seen. I went and had a complete evaluation done. He concluded that I was depressed. He told me that my extreme highs and extreme lows were consistent with bipolar illness, or manic-depression.

I didn't much like the doctor, and I didn't much like his diagnosis. I decided it was all a big mistake and that I was really "fine." I smiled politely and said I'd think about what he said. I couldn't wait to get out of his office. As I was about to leave he said, "You have to decide for yourself if you need treatment, but remember that one of the main symptoms of depression and manic depression in hard-driving, professional men like you is that you deny that you have a problem."

I left in a huff. "What does he know, anyway?" I fumed. "He's probably just trying to get more business." But I couldn't get out of my mind what he had said about denial. Carlin was supportive, but she didn't push. After a few weeks of thinking about it, I decided to see another doctor and get a second opinion. This doctor was a woman, and I liked her immediately. She was professional, but warm and accessible. I was sure she would give me a clean bill of health. After an even more extensive evaluation than I had received from the first doctor, her concluding words were almost exactly the same as his.

This time I listened. I learned that though there are certain general characteristics of depression, we each experience it differently. I found out there were many treatment approaches, including medications, psychotherapy (she used a form of cognitive behavior therapy), herbs, exercise, and diet. She also told me about some famous people in the arts who had suffered from depression or manic-depression, including Emily Dickinson, T. S. Eliot, Victor Hugo, Mark Twain, Charles

Dickens, Isak Dinesen, Ralph Waldo Emerson, William Faulkner, F. Scott Fitzgerald, Ernest Hemingway, Eugene O'Neill, Herman Melville, Tennessee Williams, and William Styron.

I figured that if I had to deal with this kind of illness, I was in pretty good company. I began taking the medications Depakote and Wellbutrin, increased my exercise program, and began counseling. Slowly things began to shift. I felt less irritable and began to enjoy life more. Carlin and I began to rebuild our strained relationship. I really never knew how depressed I was until I began feeling better. As Carlin and I began to talk about our experiences, I realized that we had a lot in common, but we also had some very different experiences of depression.

Two Kinds of Depression: Magnetic and Dynamic

The general belief among researchers in the field of gender medicine is that women are much more susceptible to depression than are men. Ellen Leibenluft, M.D., author of *Gender Differences in Mood and Anxiety Disorders,* says that "the brain is a sexually dimorphic organ and that there are marked gender differences in the prevalence of psychiatric disorders. Depression is two to three times as common in women than men." Dr. Leibenluft goes on to say that "substance abuse, in contrast, is much more common in men."

I believe that depression in men is much more prevalent than many believe, but is often hidden behind such behaviors as excessive anger, substance abuse, or overwork.

Just as there are two life forces in the natural world, the outer-directed *dynamic* and the inner-directed *magnetic,* I believe there are what I call *dynamic depressions,* which are expressed by "acting out" our inner turmoil, and *magnetic depressions,* which are expressed by "acting in" our pain. Based on my own findings over the last 37 years, I believe that men are more likely to experience dynamic depressions and women are more likely to experience magnetic depressions.

Women often express their depression by blaming themselves. Men often express their depression by blaming others—their wives, bosses, the economy, the government—anyone or anything *but* themselves. This was true in my own life. It wasn't until I recognized that my irritability, anger, and assigning blame were manifestations of depression that I was finally able to ask for help and receive treatment.

"Girls, and later women, tend to internalize pain," says psychotherapist Terrence Real. "They blame themselves and draw distress into themselves. Boys, and later men, tend to externalize pain; they are more likely to feel victimized by others and to discharge distress through action."

After 37 years of observing depression in its various forms, I developed a quiz that can help us better understand the different ways depression can manifest itself. I have come to the conclusion that depression is just as common in males as it is in females. The reason we haven't been aware of that fact is that we have focused most of our attention on the magnetic depressions and have neglected the dynamic depressions.

ACTION OPTION

Determine Your Kind of Depression

Take the following quiz to see if you tend toward magnetic depression or dynamic depression.

1. I tend to blame myself for my problems.
2. I often feel sad, worried, or worthless.
3. I often feel anxious and afraid.
4. I do my best to be nice to people.
5. When I feel hurt, I often withdraw.
6. I often feel I was born to fail.
7. I often feel slowed down and nervous.
8. I sleep a lot when I am under stress.
9. I have trouble setting good boundaries with others.
10. I often feel guilty for what I do.
11. I feel uncomfortable receiving praise.
12. I sometimes think I have a fear of success.
13. I need to blend in to feel safe.
14. I use food, friends, and "love" when I am feeling down.
15. I believe my problems would improve if only I could be a better ______ (husband, father, friend, coworker, etc.).
16. I often wonder if I am giving enough love.

If you find you have five or more of the symptoms listed above, you tend toward magnetic depression.

1. When things go wrong in my life I tend to blame others.
2. I often feel angry, irritable, and agitated.
3. I tend to feel suspicious and guarded.
4. I am often hostile even though I don't always show it.
5. When I feel hurt, I often get angry and judgmental.
6. I often feel the world was set up to fail me.
7. I tend to be restless and suspicious.
8. I often have great difficulty sleeping.
9. People tell me I am often pushy.
10. I sometimes feel ashamed for who I am.
11. I feel frustrated if I am not receiving enough praise, though I don't show it.
12. I have a real fear of failure.
13. I need to feel like the "top dog" to feel safe.
14. I use alcohol, TV sports, and sex when I am feeling down.
15. I believe my problems would improve if only my_____ (wife, children, friends, or coworkers) would treat me better.
16. I often wonder if I am getting enough love.

If you find you have five or more of the symptoms listed above, you tend toward dynamic depression.

Most people who tend toward depression have symptoms of both magnetic and dynamic depression, though one type tends to predominate. Because we have tended to focus more attention on the magnetic, or "sad," depressions, the dynamic, or "angry," depressions have often gone untreated. If symptoms cause you considerable discomfort or concern you may want to talk to a mental health professional.

Understanding Dynamic Depression in Men

I lead a group at our health clinic for men who have been referred to the court for domestic violence. On the surface, these are the last guys you'd suspect of being depressed. They laugh a lot, would usually be seen as the life of the party, and never appear sad or hurt. They are boisterous and loud. They have been heavy drinkers and most grew up in families where there was a great deal of violence. When I ask what got them in trouble, their stories are surprisingly similar. Jerry told me:

> We'd been out partying. Sharon was paying more attention to one of my friends than I thought she should and I demanded that we leave early. When we got home we got into a fight. I'm not even sure what it was about. It quickly got out of control, and Sharon said she was calling her girlfriend to come pick her up. "I've had it with your jealousy," she said. "I'm out of here."
>
> I felt panicked and enraged. When she went to make the call, I pulled the phone out of the wall. I just wanted to talk about things. I didn't want her to leave. When she ran out the door I grabbed her by the arm. "Get your hands off me," she screamed and was totally out of control. She pulled away and got in our car. By then I was out of control. I kicked out the headlights.
>
> Someone must have called the cops because the next thing I knew they had me handcuffed. The last thing I remember before they took me away was pleading with Sharon not to leave. What a mess, what a goddamned mess, I kept thinking. How could this have happened?

What the incidents these men related have in common is that they are usually triggered by the woman's desire to leave a situation she feels is dangerous and the man's attempt to keep her close. Alcohol or other drugs are often involved. The men appear enraged on the surface, but underneath there is a rising panic. And they are almost always confused. They often truly don't understand what happened.

When I'd read about the violence some of the guys in the group have been involved in I created an image in my mind that I would meet some kind of unfeeling, sociopathic, Jack the Ripper character. Instead I meet with guys who, once you get to know them, are overwhelmed with feelings and fears of loss. Rather than heartless Jack the Rippers they remind me more of depressed Peter Pans longing to find their place in a world that seems to be passing them by.

Rather than being without feeling, they seem to be overwhelmed by their feelings. Unable to express their sadness, fear, loss, worry, anxiety, hopelessness, and helplessness, they hold it all in until it finally explodes in anger and rage. We know that depression is often seen as anger turned inward. It shouldn't surprise us that anger is often an expression of depression turned outward.

Wired to Worry: A Major Source of Stress

Recent research on brain functioning has shown that depression is one of several mood disorders that has toxic worry at its center. According to Dr. Edward M. Hallowell, "People need to know how much we now understand about the treatable conditions that involve worry—such as depression, panic disorder, obsessive-compulsive disorder, generalized anxiety disorder, post-traumatic stress disorder, and attention deficit disorder."

One of the recent findings shows that there may be a genetic susceptibility to worry. A study published in the prestigious journal *Science* linked a certain gene to individuals who are prone to anxiety, pessimism, and negative thinking. The gene involved was isolated and found to be a short version of what in other people is a longer gene—specifically, the SLC6A4 gene on chromosome 17q12.

On the other side of the "worry coin" are the people who don't worry enough. These are the people in denial. Their world may be falling apart. They are eating poorly and out of shape. They are having chest pains and trouble breathing. Their wives are about to leave because "he never talks to me. All he does is drink beer and watch TV." But these guys just say to themselves, "Don't worry, be happy."

Worry alerts us to danger and lets us know that something isn't right in our world. The key to success in life isn't to avoid worrying, but to know when to worry and how to do it well. I remember worrying that I wouldn't be a good father, that I wouldn't be able to support my family. My father's old failures kept me awake at night. I worked hard at getting and keeping jobs. I worked hard to make good money. But I still worried.

One day I woke up and realized that I was still worrying about supporting my family long after I had already succeeded. My five children were grown and on their own. My wife had her own career and was quite capable of supporting herself. We had all the comforts of home and no serious wants. I chuckled when I realized I had continued running a race long after I had crossed the finish line. I realized that some worry kept me going when I might have become discouraged and quit, but too much just sours your stomach and keeps you pushing long after the goal has been met.

Not only does excessive worry sour the stomach, it may also burn the brain. When we are under a great deal of pressure our worry reflex takes over and can actually affect the workings of the brain. It seems that some people are more susceptible than others. Those who carry the "worry gene" may have less of the brain chemical serotonin. That's why antidepressant medications that block the re-uptake of serotonin can be of help to men and women who are vulnerable.

Some believe that excessive worry is a result of our genetic heritage. Others believe it is a result of environmental stress. In truth, it is both. There is always a continuing interplay between how we are programmed by our genes and the way in which our world influences our beliefs and behaviors. We are beginning to recognize that our genetic heritage has a greater influence on us than we had thought.

We all know people who have had a great deal of trauma in their lives, but seem to handle it well. We also know people whose lives seem relatively free of such trauma, but are often overwhelmed by life's ups and downs. Dealing with stress effectively may have less to do with a person's character than with his or her inborn brain chemistry.

Most men are raised to believe that they can control their emotions. If they feel down, they should just be able to "snap out of it." If they are overwhelmed they should just be able to "get it together." But we now know it isn't as easy as that. Though we are not the victims of the genetics that affect our brain chemistry, it isn't easy to change. It may require medications, therapy that reprograms our thinking, and a new kind of diet and exercise regimen.

Why Do Grown Men Act and Feel Like Boys?

One of the core issues I hear from men in midlife is that deep inside they don't really feel a strong sense of male identity. This comes from the hidden shame that most of us are afraid to admit, even to ourselves. It often leads to the excessive striving and worry that causes so much stress in our lives. "I spent most of my life trying to be the kind of man my father would be proud of, but I never felt like I made it," said Richard, a 56-year-old school principal and father of three grown children. "When I was young I worked long hours and tried to bed as many beautiful women as I could, but that didn't make me feel like a man. In my 30s and 40s I tried to be a good family man, make enough money to have a nice house, send my kids to college, and help my wife start her interior design business. Now I'm in my 50s and I've done everything right, but I still feel like there's something missing."

For many of us what was missing was a good role model of a father who was strong, loving, gentle, involved, playful, passionate. Too many of us grew up with absent fathers—absent through divorce, illness, overwork, or early death. With our isolated nuclear families, most of us did not have grandfathers, uncles, cousins, neighbors, and townsmen to provide modeling. Rather than having the experience of growing up in the presence of mature men, most of us had to make it up in our minds or from the unrealistic sitcom characters we grew up watching on TV.

Trying to Be the Opposite of a Woman

What most of us did have was a model for being female. We learned it from our mothers, older sisters, aunts, schoolteachers, and nurses. If we didn't have a clear picture of what a man was, maybe we could develop an identity in reverse by being the opposite of a woman. I remember hundreds of instances growing up where I was told that to be a proper male, I should not act like a girl: "Come on, throw that ball with some fire, not like a girl." "Stop crying, only girls cry." "You're so short, you probably should have been a girl." "Be tough, don't be a sniffling little sister."

For better or worse, girls learn directly about being feminine. For most boys being masculine is much less direct. Being male has more to do with *not* being female. Males are taught early on not to act feminine. In a thousand ways we are taught not to cry or be

- Weak
- Soft
- Tender
- Beautiful
- Passive
- Receptive
- Sweet
- Apologetic
- Unsure of ourselves

This is a poor way to build a male identity. A foundation based not on who we are but on who we aren't is forever shaky. Since as human males we have all the qualities of a full human being, to deny half these qualities limits our humanity. And since we are not given a positive direction to move toward—positive qualities of masculinity—we feel adrift in fear and uncertainty.

At midlife we can no longer fulfill an identity based on what we are not. Either we reclaim our full humanity or we spend our later years acting like aging children, clinging to a male identity that, like the emperor's clothing, is illusory. At the core of male shame and depression is the sense that at the center of our being, where our sense of manhood ought to be, is a black hole. Filling that hole with the richness of male identity, not the dross of pseudomanhood, is one of the main tasks of midlife.

Fear and Stress over Job Losses

Many of us blame ourselves when we lose our jobs. If we have a job, we are constantly worried about losing it. For most of us our identity, our pride, our passion, even our sexuality, is tied up with our work. If we are not working, we don't feel fully alive—not a whole man, not fully human.

Yet recent economic trends have left millions of us permanently unemployed or underemployed. Tens of millions of jobs have been erased in North America in the last 20 years, according to a *New York Times* analysis of Labor Department statistics. In the last 20 years North America has transformed itself into a postindustrial society. The result has been good for big business and bad for men and their families.

College-educated men over 45 have seen our yearly pay descend by 18 percent over the last five years. As America's economy becomes even more high tech and specialized, traditional blue-collar male jobs (i.e., factory, construction, and transportation) have become scarce. During the 1980s the number of men who were working full time year-round declined by over 10 percent. By 1991 the number of men working full time year-round was declining by 1.2 million each year.

Nearly three-quarters of all households have had a close encounter with layoffs since 1980, according to a poll by the *New York Times*. We once thought the high-tech industry was the place to be for secure work. We now know that there is no greater job security working for a dot-com company than for a traditional company.

In her excellent book *Stiffed: The Betrayal of the American Man,* feminist author Susan Faludi concludes that the male stress, shame, depression, and violence are not just a problem of individual men, but a product of the social betrayal of men that occurred after World War II. In the dream of postwar America, we would all follow in the footsteps of our fathers and enter a world of work that was secure and would allow us to bestow on our families the benefits of an affluent society.

"Implicit in all of this," says Faludi, "was a promise of loyalty, a guarantee to the new man of tomorrow that his company would never fire him, his wife would never leave him, and the team he rooted for would never pull up stakes. Instead, the average man found his father was an absent father, the job market had no place for him, women were ashamed of his inability to make a decent living, and even his favorite sports team abandoned him."

The biggest betrayal, as I found out with my father, was the way postwar America destroyed our economic base. When we lose our jobs, or are in constant fear of losing our jobs, at the same time we are going through midlife, it can be devastating.

Many of us take out our frustrations in violent ways, directed at ourselves or those around us. We become impotent with rage. Unable to assume our positions as men, more and more of us are left in limbo. Just when we feel we should be passing on the fruits of our success to the next generation, being a man of pride and substance, we are cut off at the knees.

Instead of being able to give blessings and wisdom to our adult sons and daughters, we feel we have reverted to acting like children ourselves. Instead of feeling we can pass on the fruits of our labor, we find that our tree no longer bears fruit. Instead of becoming an elder in the family and the community, we find we have become aging children. We long to feel that we are men of substance, but instead feel that our manhood is only skin deep.

These are hard truths for most of us to accept. Yet the first step in healing is to recognize and understand the depth of our emotional pain. Once we can accept the fact that we are hurting, we can take the next steps in the healing process.

CHAPTER 11

Healing Our Emotional Selves

People will do anything to be enlightened except give up their suffering.

—Gurdjieff

Our Hidden Emotions

From the time we were small boys we were taught to hide our emotional pain. Even as adults, we carry this emotional repression. I remember the day I heard that my father had died. I was visiting a friend of a friend I did not know very well. My wife had called to let me know. I hung up the phone and smiled. Though I was crying inside I felt embarrassed to let a virtual stranger know how I was feeling. I only let myself show any feelings once I was alone, and even then I felt I had to keep my emotions under control.

However, our emotions have a way of sneaking through the cracks of our well-built defenses. There are often signs from inside that everything is not quite right. We

- Feel a vague sense of dis-ease
- Feel irritable and angry
- Feel bored with life
- Want to run away and start over

For many of us, healing our physical bodies is hard enough. Healing our emotional bodies may seem like an impossible task. I hope the following steps will make it easier for you.

1. Accept the reality of your emotional pain.

Look back over the stories, ideas, and concepts you have read in the previous chapter and pay attention to those that stand out for you.

"Standing out" may be something that resonates with you. Something inside you says, "Yes, that feels right to me. I've experienced something like that before." I felt like that as soon as I read the material on worry.

On the other hand, it may be something that you protest against: "No, no, no. That's not me. I'm not anything like that." Looking back, I can see that is how I responded to my depression. Look for the concepts about which you may protest too much. I've learned the hard way that when I'm defensive about looking at something, it is often because there is some truth in what is there.

Sometimes finding what stands out in our emotional life is very vague and may not seem like it has anything to do with our emotions at all. I remember going to a doctor for a full year to treat prostatitis, an inflammation of the prostate gland. I was experiencing burning when I urinated and went to a urologist for help. He was sure it could be easily treated with antibiotics, which he prescribed. When one didn't work, he tried another one.

I was not getting any better and finally went to another doctor. After giving me a complete physical examination, he asked if I was under any stress in my life. Somewhat reluctantly, I talked about the communication problems I was having with my wife, particularly about sex.

What did this unusual doctor give me? He prescribed drinking a gallon of water a day to flush out all the medications I had been taking. Then he gave me some suggestions about improving our communication about sex. My problems were gone within two weeks. I learned a lot about the ways our suppressed emotions can express themselves in physical symptoms.

2. Learn to name your emotions.

For most of us, learning how to express our emotions is like learning to speak Greek, Russian, or Chinese. We don't even know where to begin. Once we become aware of our emotional pain, we need to learn to name our emotions. How many times have we been asked, usually by a woman, "What are you feeling?" Most of the time we're not even aware we are feeling anything. When we answer "Nothing," she is incredulous and frustrated.

Even when we know we are feeling something we don't know how to name it. Our emotional vocabulary is limited. I've found it helpful to start with four basic emotions that I call mad, sad, glad, and afraid. To keep our emotional life in good shape, we need to be able to begin to understand our feelings. When I'm not sure what I feel, I go down the list.

- Am I feeling any irritation or anger?
- Am I feeling sad or down?
- Am I feeling happy and upbeat?
- Am I feeling anxious or afraid?

Some are more skilled at feeling and expressing some emotions than others. I grew up in a family in which sadness was acceptable, but anger was never expressed. My friend Joe experienced the opposite: "Everyone yelled at everyone in our family. Dad screamed at Mom. Mom passed it on to the kids. We kids fought with each other. But if anyone acted like they were afraid or started to cry, he would be taunted mercilessly."

3. Practice expressing the range of your emotions.

I find that most people differ in which emotions they most commonly express first when they are under pressure. One group has anger on the surface. Another group most often expresses hurt feelings first. Men more often are the ones who more easily experience anger, but have more difficulty expressing hurt. Women tend to be the opposite.

But here's what's interesting. When we look below the surface of men's anger we often find the sadness and hurt. Underneath women's hurt, they often hold a great deal of anger. Think about which emotion is on the surface for you. If you find you get angry easily, learn how to express your sadness and hurt. If you are better at expressing your hurt, learn to express your anger.

When we continue to delve even deeper, we find that under the anger and hurt, there is often a great deal of fear. "This was a revelation to me," said Frank, a patient who I had seen over a period of many months. "I started counseling because my wife said she would leave me if I didn't get control of my anger. I didn't think counseling would help. We'd been married for nearly 30 years and she did a lot of things that made me mad. Plus I've been trying to control my anger all my life and nothing has ever worked."

After one of Frank's angry outbursts in my office, I asked him to tell me how hurt he really felt. "I immediately got tears in my eyes," Frank recalled. "I had no idea I was feeling hurt. I felt so sad that our marriage wasn't working, but until that moment I never realized I had any other feelings than irritation and anger."

A number of sessions later I asked Frank how afraid he felt. "I really *was* afraid, but I never wanted to admit it," he confided. "When Marcia and I first got together I was amazed that she would really like a guy like me. I've always worried that she'd find someone who was less angry, more stable, better looking. When I finally let out the fear, it was like a weight had been lifted off of me."

The real help for men who have chronic anger is not to try to control it more effectively. What we really need is to learn to express our hurt and fear more directly. After Frank learned to feel and express a greater range of feelings, I had a session with him and his wife. "It's like a miracle," Marcia told us. "He's like the man I remember from our courting days. I can feel his gentleness and warmth now, which had somehow gotten lost."

I looked at Frank. He was nodding his head and smiling with a calm, almost sweet look of pleasure and peace. I asked Frank how he was feeling. He chuckled as he answered. "Two years ago I wouldn't have even known I was feeling anything. A year ago I would have known something was going on inside me, but wouldn't have known what it was. Now . . . now, I'm feeling warm . . . caring . . . proud . . . joyful . . . and loving."

Frank was looking at his wife. He reached out to hold her hand. Both had tears in their eyes. They had gotten to the fourth level of feeling. He had gotten underneath the anger at level one, the hurt at level two, and the fear at level three. He was now experiencing the wonderful feeling of joy and love at level four. I would go so far as to say that anger, hurt, and fear are expressions of love. They are just incomplete expressions. Each feeling is trying to take us to the next level.

Rather than try to control one feeling we may not like, we need to learn to express a wider range of emotions. When a man or a woman tells me they don't feel love in their relationship, I know for certain that anger, hurt, and fear are being suppressed.

The way I've experienced this in my life is that it's felt like my feelings have become frozen. I feel cold and lifeless, and I'm sure I come across as distant and cool. Once I get my feelings flowing and the anger, hurt, or fear I've been holding back begins to thaw, the natural love that is inside has a chance to express itself.

4. Recognize that men are the more emotionally sensitive sex.

One of the major complaints I hear in marriages that are in trouble is that the man won't talk about what's going on or how he feels. Dr. John Gottman, one of the world's experts on human relationships, calls this male tendency to withhold feelings "stonewalling." In his book *Why Marriages Succeed or Fail,* he shows how destructive this can be to a relationship.

What Gottman has demonstrated, through careful experimentation in his marriage lab, is the *reason* so many of us stonewall. It isn't because we are less emotional than women. Its because we are *overwhelmed* by our emotions. Withdrawal is our way of protecting ourselves from becoming flooded by our feelings.

"Our research has shown that men are more likely to become stonewallers than are women," says Gottman. "The reason, I believe, may be biological. Men tend to be more physiologically overwhelmed than women by marital tension—for example, during confrontations a man's pulse rate is more likely to rise, along with his blood pressure. Therefore, men may feel a greater, perhaps instinctive, need to flee from intense conflict with their spouse in order to protect their health," Gottman concludes.

If a man is flooded by his feelings he will tend to withdraw if he can. I have found that many angry confrontations between men and women are a result of the man trying to withdraw and the woman continuing to try and get him to talk and respond.

I remember one such extreme confrontation in my own life. There had been a great deal of tension between my second wife, Anne, and myself over a period of many months. We would get into long arguments, and I would feel continually panicked and exhausted. I felt totally overwhelmed—in Gottman's terms, flooded—and finally retreated into the bedroom and closed the door.

I felt my heart beginning to slow down and the pressure in my head starting to subside when the door burst open and my wife came striding into the room. "Don't you dare walk out when I'm talking to you," she screamed. "We've got to talk about these things. You can't keep running away from them."

Immediately my heart began to race and my face got hot with frustration and anger. I felt trapped. "Just back off, OK?" I almost pleaded. "Let's talk about it later. I just can't keep on any more tonight." I felt my attention narrow, almost like my vision was closing down.

I knew if she didn't back away I would lose it. I'd never hit her or been violent in any way. I always saw myself as a peaceful, reasonable man who wouldn't hurt a fly. But I felt I was being pushed beyond my limit. I think she felt my rising panic and sensed that I was losing control.

She started out the door, but then turned back toward me. She kept coming until she was inches from me and began to scream in my face, "Goddamn you, you bastard." As her words spewed out, she began pounding her index finger into my chest. I felt like I was being touched with a hot poker. I felt my control dissolve.

In the split seconds when she began screaming again and pounding my chest, I totally lost control. I felt my fist come back. It was like it was moving in slow motion, disconnected from the rest of my body, moving with a will of its own. All I could see was her raging face, full of venom. I just wanted her to stop. I knew I couldn't stop. I was too far gone. I had lost control. The smoldering embers, so long kept under control, had burst into flame and threatened to consume everything in sight. I moved forward and she backed up.

As my fist flew through the air I knew destruction was in its path and that my life would never be the same again. My fist flashed past her head on a path for the wall. There was so much frustration, fear, and rage built up in me I was sure I would go right through the wall. I saw my arm coming out the other side of the house and the entire structure collapsing around us.

Instead I was stopped by a stud standing guard behind the wall. My fist did not go through it. I did not bring the house down. Instead, I heard the bones break as my hand crumpled. I looked down at it as it started immediately to swell. My wife stared at me, a mix of gratitude and fear showing on her pale face. At least I had gotten her to shut up, I thought. We were silent as she drove me to the emergency room. The shock had not worn off, and the pain had not yet begun.

When the doctor finally saw me and the X rays were complete, he wanted to know what the other guy looked like. "I haven't seen breaks like these since I doctored boxers when I was in the army," he said. I just shrugged my shoulders. I found it ironic that when a woman comes into the emergency room with even a bruise, doctors are alert to the possibility of domestic violence. When a man comes in with broken bones, they assume he's been in a fight with another man.

The next day, after I had awakened from the anesthesia, the surgeon told me the operation had gone as well as could be expected. Six bones in my right hand had been badly broken. It would take months to heal and years before I would know how much motion would return.

As I write this, it has been nearly 25 years since my suppressed anger burst forth. The scars remain. My hand doesn't work quite right, but I've gotten used to doing what I can do. More importantly, in the intervening years I have learned to deal with my anger and depression.

5. Heal your anger.

If you'd asked me before the "fist in the stud incident," as I have come to refer to the above experience, I would have told you that I'm not an angry man. In fact, I would have said that I hardly ever got angry.

The first step for many of us in healing our anger is to become aware that we can *feel* a great deal of anger without ever expressing it. Looking back on my life, I could see that I experienced all kinds of angry, sometimes violent thoughts, but never paid attention to them. I told myself that if I didn't act angry then I wasn't *really* angry, and that those feelings would just go away.

The truth is that they don't go away; they just bury themselves ever more deeply in our minds. They contribute to high blood pressure, stroke, heart attack, and cancer. This kind of anger is like acid; it slowly eats away at us from the inside.

To heal, we must feel. Once we can feel our anger, we can learn to express it in appropriate ways. We can move through the anger to our hurt, our fear, and finally to our feelings of love. We can talk to a trusted friend or our spouse. We can yell our anger and frustrations to the wind and the rain and let the elements cleanse us. There are many things we can do to heal our anger once we become aware of how much we are holding inside us.

A much smaller percentage of men come from angry or violent backgrounds. If you are one of these guys, your anger is never far from the surface. Your fuse is short, and you can explode at the smallest hurt or perceived put-down. You need to know that your anger is destroying you and your relationships.

I have run groups for guys like you over the last 25 years and have found that the main ingredient to helping you heal is to give you firm boundaries and let you know that your violence will not be tolerated—either in the group, in your home, or in your community. Once boundaries are established you need to learn self-respect and self-love. Although you may act tough, inside I know you can feel vulnerable and afraid.

I tell you that your violent behavior must stop, but I also tell you that you are a good and valuable man. In all ways, I try to treat you with respect, compassion, and caring. I know, as many do not, that it could easily be me whose anger had gotten out of control and resulted in violence. I believe we all carry that potential.

However, out of our fear and frustration as a society we are increasingly likely to punish guys like you—to lock you up and remove you from society. This is the opposite of what is needed. You do need boundaries and limits, but you also need understanding, support, and good role modeling.

Whether bottled up inside or expressed openly, anger is a problem for most men. Healing our anger can go a long way toward healing our selves and our relationships.

6. Heal your depression.

Depression is the silent killer of men. Although depression is extremely common and very treatable, few men get help. Most of us don't even recognize that we are depressed. Look back over the questionnaire on magnetic and dynamic depression in chapter 10. We often find it very difficult to see depression in ourselves.

ACTION OPTION

Explore Your Magnetic and Dynamic Depressions

Have someone you know and trust fill out the questionnaire as that person sees you. Ask him or her to be as honest as possible. Take the quiz again yourself. Write down the items you both agree upon. Notice the items your companion may have noted that you don't see in yourself. Put an X next to those items you may not be aware of but suspect you express under pressure.

As I said in discussing my own story, I had to be pulled in kicking and screaming to see the doctor. I'm sure I'm not alone in that. Most of us men hate to see a doctor, and even worse than seeing a regular doctor is going to see a "head" doctor. Many of us, me included (even though I am a mental health professional and should know better after all these years), associate going to a "shrink" with being "crazy."

Once we go, however, we find that depression is an illness just like diabetes. We're not crazy if we get our diabetes treated, and we're not crazy if we get our emotions treated. I found that many of the fears we have about seeing a therapist are unfounded.

After we've seen a health professional we will learn that depression isn't "all in our mind," that it is caused by physical changes in our brain chemistry and can be effectively treated. Over 90 percent of those coming for treatment can be helped. There are a range of treatments available, everything from the newest pharmaceutical drugs to herbal remedies that have been used for thousands of years.

At our clinic, we treat depression in a number of ways. We offer medications, herbs, exercise, massage, acupuncture, cognitive behavior therapy, psychotherapy, and couples counseling. We even offer employment counseling.

One of the major concerns I have heard from men, and one I had myself, was that if they go to a doctor they will be given an antidepressant. If they take an antidepressant it may have a negative effect on their sex lives, which is sure to make them more depressed. So why go at all?

I'll give you three good reasons. First, if you're depressed, there are many things we can offer other than pharmaceutical medications. We have learned that there are many ways of changing our brain chemistry. As Dr. Joel Robertson and Tom Monte, coauthors of *Natural Prozac,* remind us, "Our brain chemistry is altered by food, exercise, thoughts, emotions, and actions, as well as by drugs." If you decide not to take antidepressant medication there's likely to be something that will work well for you.

Second, although some men do experience negative sexual side effects from some of the antidepressants, most do not. You won't know which group you fall into until you try. I had one client who was taking Zoloft (an antidepressant similar to Prozac). He quickly complained that the medication was interfering with his love life. He told me the name should be changed to "No Loft." I suggested that there were other medications that could help.

Third, since depression is such a widespread problem, newer drugs are constantly coming on the market with fewer side effects. I told him about four other drugs we might try: Effexor, Serzone, Remeron, and Wellbutrin. Given his particular symptoms, we first tried Wellbutrin. He was very pleased with the results. "Not only has it helped the depression," he told me after being on the medication for three weeks, "but it has actually *helped* my sex life. The 'loft' has returned big time. My wife and I are experiencing the kind of sexual pleasure we had in earlier years. I'm glad I hung in there and kept trying."

7. Heal your emotional hypersensitivity.

For years my wife, Carlin, and I would have fights over feelings. She would often seem cold and distant to me. When I'd ask why, she would tell me she was protecting herself from my anger. This would often set me off. I'd start in a quiet tone of voice. "Be reasonable, I don't get angry that much," I'd tell her.

"Yes, you do," she'd reply. "You get angry a lot more than you think."

Now I really *was* beginning to get angry. Why is she jabbing at me? I'd think. "Damn it, if you don't want me to get angry, stop provoking me," I'd yell, even though I tried to control my outburst. She'd look at me with a mixture of disbelief and hurt. "I was just trying to be caring," she'd say. I'd look back at her with my eyes narrow and piercing. She calls it my beady-eyed look. If you call that caring, I'd say to myself, I'd rather be cared for by a pack of wild dogs. We remained stuck for a long time.

Things began to change when I started to see how sensitive I was and how easily my emotions could be triggered. I also realized that I was getting even more sensitive the older I got. I've found that a stern look, a raised eyebrow, a judgmental tone of voice can be interpreted as a put-down. Even a hug, a loving comment, or a kind look can be misinterpreted and perceived as negative.

The way I've come to see it, many of us have become emotionally hypersensitive—only we don't know it, and those around us don't know it. As a result a loving embrace "hurts like hell." A friendly pat on the back can feel like we are "being attacked." A loving comment can make us "wince with pain." Since we don't know we are hypersensitive, we are sure that those who touch us emotionally must want to hurt us. Why else would they treat us that way? Because our partners and friends don't know we are hypersensitive, they can't understand why their gestures of love are met with resistance and anger.

"You tell me you wonder why I'm angry. How do you expect me to react when you hit me in the head with a two-by-four?" I remember yelling at my wife during one of my outbursts in response to something hurtful I felt she had said to me. She looked at me in disbelief and amazement. Her response was equally unbelievable to me: "Are you kidding? I reach out to you with love and you attack me."

Once we recognize and accept our extreme emotional sensitivity, we can begin to heal. Counseling and therapy can often help us heal the old wounds from our past that have caused us to be hypersensitive. Even while we are healing from the past, knowing we are sensitive can help us reinterpret the kinds of response we get from others. Once I became aware that I was hypersensitive, I didn't feel Carlin was out to get me. I could see that she was often sending me love, but I had been unable to register it because of my emotional pain. Now I can let the love in and know I am being cared for.

Knowing that I am still somewhat sensitive, Carlin doesn't react to my occasional winces when she does or says something that she is sure is loving. Instead of withdrawing or reacting with anger, she can stay with me, sometimes tone down the level of her emotional energy just a bit, and know that I am not rejecting her.

8. Learn to go for the joy.

I have recently come to realize that I have spent a great deal of my life either in emotional pain or trying to protect myself from emotional pain. I became aware of how often my thoughts strayed to the negative. Somewhere past my 50th year I decided to change how I looked at the world. Instead of focusing on what I didn't want and how I didn't want to feel, I wanted to focus more on what I did want.

I decided I wanted more joy, fun, laughter, spontaneity, adventure, music, dance, and travel. I also began to change the way I counseled people who came to me for help. In the past, if you came to see me, I would start by asking you to tell me about your problems. That's what most therapists and doctors do. First we find out about the problem, then we try to treat it.

When I first began studying to become a therapist 37 years ago, the emphasis was on what was wrong with you and what to do to fix it. We took course after course on psychopathology and learned all the ways that people are damaged by their early childhood experiences. The practice of psychotherapy involved digging back into our early life experience to try to get at the root of what caused the damage to our psyches. Once we got to the core of things and recognized why we were so messed up, it was hoped that we would be able to take charge of our lives and become happier and better-adjusted human beings.

The problem was, this approach takes a long time, it doesn't always produce the results that it claims, and men tend to avoid it like the plague. If we ever do come for this kind of therapy, we usually don't stay for very long. I've changed the approach I use in my own life and also in what I do with my clients.

Now the first questions I'd ask you if you came to me for help are "What would you like in coming to see me? How would you like your life to be?" This sets the stage for a change in the whole atmosphere of therapy. From the very beginning we focus on the positive. I have found that we don't need to immerse ourselves in all of our life problems in order to find contentment and joy.

I also found, to my surprise, that therapy has become a lot more fun for me and those who come to me for help. Men, particularly, seemed to appreciate an approach that dealt with here-and-now issues rather than digging up old ghosts from the past. When we did look into the past, which I sometimes still found helpful, our searches were specific and time limited, and always related to helping you get where you want to go.

I also found that men started to get better quicker. I was able to empower them to see their life differently, to help them recognize that they are OK just the way they are. I began to see that they didn't need to heal their pathology, that in fact there is no pathology at all—just a life, a work in progress, with all its beautiful downs and ups, ins and outs. They begin to see just how valuable they are—not when their life gets better, not when they lose weight, not when they make more money, not when their marriage improves—but right now, right here.

I have found that helping you improve your life works much better when we start from a position that you are a perfect you, not a you that is sick and needs to be changed. Like a rosebud, we will grow and change over time; but at any given time, we are perfect just the way we are. Focusing on the positive in ourselves, and in what we want in the world, seems to work a lot better than focusing on what is wrong and what we don't want.

There's an old saying that what we focus on expands. It makes sense to me that if we want more pathology, pain, and misery in our lives, it will help to focus on the past, on trauma, and our present state of unhappiness. However, if we want more health, pleasure, and joy, it will serve us to focus on the future, on wellness, and on the glory of who we are at our best and our brightest.

When I first started using this approach I thought, "Things can't get better just by looking on the bright side. That's just wishful thinking, Pollyanna, pie in the sky." I thought of my hippie friends in the 1960s who spent their days and nights staying stoned and thinking good thoughts for the future. Many of them are dead now, dead from drugs or despair. Others are busy catching up for lost time, working their butts off to save enough money to survive when they retire.

To paraphrase an old saying, there's more to health than positive thinking and there's more to positive thinking than positive thinking. When I keep focused on what I want in life, on the positive feelings I want, it brings about positive actions. It also helps me focus on the larger issues related to my life's calling, the focus of chapter 12.

Finding Someone with a Similar Story

I have had many people tell me that hearing someone else talk about his or her own life was extremely healing. When we hear someone else's story we are often able to empathize in a way that allows us to open our hearts to our own experiences. Sometimes we are in the presence of the person who opens his or her life to us; at other times the experience occurs at a distance.

An important person who spoke to me through her writing was Kay Redfield Jamison. I had known of her as one of the preeminent professionals in the field of mental health. She is a professor of psychiatry at the Johns Hopkins School of Medicine and the co-author of the standard medical text on manic-depressive illness. What I didn't know until I read her memoir, *An Unquiet Mind,* was that she, too, suffered from serious mood disorders and resisted medications and treatment for a long time.

Her early experiences seemed to mirror my own. She told of times when she felt utterly alone. Seeing the animated conversations of others only made her feel more withdrawn. She would drift down into loneliness and despair or up into agitation and irritation. She said she was not easy to be around, but had convinced herself that she was normal, surely no worse than colleagues and friends.

I knew exactly what she meant. It sounded like she was telling my story. If another professional of her standing could admit she had emotional problems, maybe I could, too. It made it easier for me to seek and accept help. Whenever I start feeling that I don't need help, that I can handle my problems myself, I reread her book. It always reminds me to be humble and keeps me on a healthy path.

Is there anyone's story that gives you strength when you are feeling down? If so, continue to allow those experiences to nourish your emotional well-being. If not, seek out a person through his or her writings or face-to-face and let that person's emotional healing give you the strength to heal.

CHAPTER 12

From Career to Calling: Finding Our Spirit

Try not to become a man of success, rather become a man of value.

—Albert Einstein

"I'M NOT SURE WHERE I'm going with my life," says Joseph, a good-looking 46-year-old man who looks a good deal like Tom Cruise.

> On one level I feel like I have it all. I'm married to a wonderful woman. Our children are nearly grown. I've been very successful as a business consultant. We have friends and extended family who we enjoy. But on the other hand I feel lost and alone. I wonder whether I've wasted my years, if I've really contributed anything of value.
>
> I look at my wife, Karen, who I love dearly, and all I can see are the flaws in her appearance and her behavior. I don't feel turned on to her sexually in the same way I did in the past. Her body doesn't excite me as it once did, but I find myself almost obsessively attracted to younger women who I seem to see everywhere.

Joseph raises his eyes with a sad and imploring look on his face. Joseph is like so many men I have seen between 40 and 55. He is in a transition phase of his life, but he doesn't know it. He feels lost and alone, but he thinks the main problem is with women. He's looking for a deeper meaning in life, but he's looking outside himself.

Some of us do make mistakes and choose the wrong partner, but at this age we are often looking for our lost selves. What few men realize is that we are looking for love in all the wrong places. What they really seek will never be found in the arms of another woman, or in any other person.

In the first part of our lives many of us fell in love, got married, and had children before we really knew what kind of career would make us happy. A great deal of our pain comes from our decision to find a partner to join in our lives before we had a clear sense of where we wanted to go.

Now, in the second half of our lives, we must choose again. The old desires remain strong. As Joseph found, it is very easy to start seeing all the flaws in the woman we are with and go looking for another kind of woman to make us happy. We tell ourselves we want a woman who is __________. (Fill in the blank: More understanding; sexier; prettier; more interested in us; career oriented; family oriented; more nurturing; kinder.)

The truth is, we won't find what we are looking for in *any* woman, no matter how perfect she seems. What we are searching for at this stage of our lives is to finish our career and begin our calling.

My Career Story

I have been pursuing a career as a psychotherapist for over 35 years. I love what I do, and I feel I have had a wonderful career. Looking back, I realize I kind of fell into this line of work. Growing up, I was attracted to business. Since my father was gone by the time I was six, I modeled my early career interests after what I thought my mother wanted me to do.

At first I thought I wanted to be a doctor, and in college I majored in biology. I did well in college, graduated high in my class, and was accepted into the medical school at the University of California, San Francisco, where I finally discovered that I wasn't cut out to be a doctor. Among other things, I kept fainting at the sight of blood. I also found that the competition was cutthroat and no one praised me for knowing all the bones in the body. I left and enrolled in the School of Social Welfare at the University of California, Berkeley. If you'd asked me why, and if I had been willing to tell you the truth, I would have admitted that I needed to go somewhere so that I wouldn't have to leave the country or go to jail. The Vietnam War was in full swing at that time, a war I didn't believe in and couldn't bring myself to join in any way.

It was at Berkeley that my career began to come together. I found I liked to help people, and I seemed to be pretty good at it. I had two wonderful teachers whose example made me want to be a social worker who practiced psychotherapy.

They were both talented in working one-on-one with a client, but they also taught us that we had to be aware that our clients lived in the real world. We had to understand their family constellation, race, ethnic background, and level of poverty or economic status, as well as what drugs (including caffeine, nicotine, and alcohol) they used to deal with life's stresses.

Over the years I developed a very successful career. It enabled me to make money at something I loved to do. I found a woman to marry me, and we had children. I bought a nice house, and we raised our children in it. We had our ups and downs, as I mentioned before, and eventually divorced.

I kept my career going while I tried my best to maintain a relationship with my children. I didn't know it would be so difficult. I thought, being a therapist, that I knew all the right things to keep a marriage working well. I learned that being a therapist didn't protect my marriage. I thought that being a therapist would, at least, allow my wife and me to separate on good terms. It definitely didn't help.

Looking back, I can see that I was so immersed and overwhelmed in developing my career that I didn't pay enough attention to my family. I wish I had had the wisdom to get my career well established *before* looking for the woman to join me. Failing that, I wish I had waited to have children. They all suffered because of my lack of vision. But back then, I could only see what I could see. As they say, I'm older than that now.

ACTION OPTION

Examine Your Career Path

Get out a piece of paper and title it "Career Development." Write down the highlights of your career path. Pay particular attention to the people that influenced your choices and how you felt about your various jobs. Write about what aspects you particularly enjoyed and which ones you did not like. Finally, write about your feelings of fulfillment at this time of life.

The Seeds of Our Calling

I remember when I first became aware that there was a difference between my career and my calling. I was at a men's retreat, still feeling slightly guilty that I was doing something without my wife and family. One of the exercises involved looking deeply inside us to help discover our purpose for the second half of our lives.

We thought back to when we were children and the challenges we had faced. I thought of my father's illness and my desire to do something in the helping professions. Think back on your own early experiences. What were the challenges you faced and overcame? Could they be related to your calling in life?

We were also asked to think of things that brought us joy. We were told to pay particular attention to the time period between 9 and 12 years old. For many of us, it was a time when we were at the pinnacle of our childhood powers and before we began the search for sex and finding the right woman. I thought of the times I spent with my buddies. We'd fight and roughhouse, but we were very close.

I remembered Jack, Lester, and David. We'd play, share songs, talk about sports or what we wanted to do when we grew up, but mostly we just gloried in being ourselves and being together. Every day was an adventure. Night was a time to play in the dark. We never wanted to come inside. I remembered we painted our football white so we could continue playing when it was dark and still see the ball.

ACTION OPTION

Delve into the Dreams of Your Calling

Get out a sheet of paper and title it "9 to 12." Write down the highlights of what you remember during those years. Pay particular attention to any hopes and dreams you had about your future. If you had some, write them down and also detail how you felt about the possibility of fulfilling those dreams. Did you get encouragement from those around you, or did they tell you that your dreams were frivolous or unattainable? Did you have anyone you shared your dreams with? Find someone you feel close to and share your memories.

When it came time for me to write my purpose, what came out was that *I wanted to dedicate my life to helping men live long and well.* I wanted to help males of all ages to fulfill the best of who we can be throughout our lives. I wanted our relationships with our fathers, mothers, wives, children, grandchildren, friends, colleagues, communities, and planet to be healthy, joyful, and as nourishing as possible.

As soon as I said my purpose out loud, I had a shame and guilt attack. Who was I, after all, to think I could help men in all our relationships? And what about women? Would I stop seeing women as clients? What would women think? What would my wife think? What would my *mother* think?

I realized that I had always been drawn to helping men but was afraid to acknowledge it. It never bothered me when women said they wanted to work with other women. Why did it take me so long to accept that my purpose involved helping men?

"Each of us is born with an innate character, the 'daimon' or 'spirit,'" says psychologist James Hillman, "that calls us to what we are meant to be." We feel the pull of this spirit throughout our lives, but during the first half it is often buried by the many "shoulds" we live with: I should be a good boy, husband, man, father. I should be responsible and make a good living. I should do what the woman wants me to do. I should *not* do what the woman wants me to do. I should be strong and silent.

In many ways I have found that in the first part of our lives we are living out what our parents wanted us to be or rebelling against what our parents wanted us to be. Sometime between 35 and 45 we feel the first strong stirrings of our true spirit beginning to assert itself. If we listen to it, our daimon will guide our lives in the second half and allow us to feel the peace and fulfillment that comes from expressing our true self in the world. If we stick to our old patterns and deny the calling of our spirit, we become frozen and sick. We begin to lose our vital energy and ultimately begin to go downhill and become despondent and emotionally numb.

This is a frightening time for us. Whatever life we have achieved or failed to achieve in the first half is at least familiar. When we begin hearing the call of our spirit, it can be terrifying. Am I going to have to give up all I've achieved? Will I have to start over at a new job? Is there really something more important than what I've been doing all these years? What if I go after it and I fail? Will I be left all alone?

It's no wonder so many of us would rather avoid these questions and go back to an earlier time. But avoidance is dangerous. I have seen too many men literally work themselves to death in their later years rather than slow down enough to get in touch with their true calling.

I've also seen men move into the second half with no sense of purpose. We find ourselves awash in confusion, doubt, and despair. Studies show that lack of purpose in life is one of the foremost predictors of fatal heart attacks. We also know that as men age our suicide risk increases dramatically.

These problems don't seem to occur in societies in which elder males have important roles. It may help us to think more about our calling if we examine some of the traditional roles that have motivated men throughout the ages.

Reclaiming Traditional Roles for Men in the Second Half of Life

We often think of modern society as bringing us more of the good things in life. There is no doubt that we live longer than we have lived throughout most of human history. But there is also more stress and conflict. Young males are becoming more and more violent, and our attempts to control them by threatening them and locking them up are clearly ineffective.

We have not done a very good job of passing on wisdom about how to live well to the younger generation. Young males, particularly, seem to be having a difficult time receiving the role modeling that allows them to grow into responsible adults. In teaching young men to embrace the values of adult society, we have a lot to learn from premodern societies.

There are a number of critical roles that older men are encouraged to embrace and express in these societies. These include the roles of peacemaker, spirit guide, and male mentor. Anthropologist Austin Shelton describes the roles of the Nsukka Ibo men of Nigeria: "The older man reaches a stage of life in which he leaves farming and manual labor to the young, on the grounds that he must now devote his energies to more important matters—maintaining order and justice in the clan, keeping his people under the protection of God and the ancestors, and teaching the young the correct ways of human relationships."

The Role of Peacemaker

In traditional societies throughout Africa, for example, one of the prime roles of older men is as peacemaker. Anthropologist Paul

Spencer found this role is prevalent among the Samburu of eastern Africa (an offshoot tribe of the bellicose Masai), as well as the Zulu, the Nyakyusa, and the Lele of central Africa.

They recognize that the young men must express their aggression, but they also recognize that the role of elder males is to channel and control it. "While the old men of these tribes might recognize that the intemperate young man is the best vessel for the collective aggression of the group," says Dr. David Gutmann, a social scientist, "they also recognize that this aggression must be physically removed from the vulnerable precincts of the intimate community."

One of the real tragedies of our modern society is that this role has become diminished. Many of us have become too frightened of young males to help them channel their aggression into constructive action. As a result, we are building more prisons to house them. What they really need is the active involvement of older men as peacemakers.

There are a number of programs, for instance, where veterans talk to young men about the realities of war. The vets can identify with the younger men's youthful zeal to prove their masculinity and act in heroic ways. Young men can often identify with an elder male who has proven himself in battle. Many can tell the truth about war and killing in such a way that young men can really hear it. Young men learn that there are better ways to develop a sense of masculine pride than by killing others.

There are older men who go into areas of the world where young men are killing each other and help both sides learn to see their common humanity. Young men are hungry to have such guidance. And you don't have to go into foreign war zones to be a peacemaker. Young males are killing and dying in every community in the country. Find out how you can get involved.

Many young men are looking to test themselves and display their courage under pressure. I practice a martial art called aikido. It originated in Japan and has become popular throughout the world. It is a superb practice for learning to stay calm under pressure and to defend yourself in all situations.

My teacher told the story of a young man who had come to the dojo. He was a street kid from the inner city and told the instructor he wanted to learn how to kill. Rather than throwing the young man out of the building or telling him aikido was a peaceful practice, he invited the young man in. The instructor, an ex-marine who had been an instructor with the Special Forces, told the young man that he could teach him how to kill.

He told him that it would take a year and that he had to come to the dojo at least once a week for that time. If he missed a session, he would have to start over again. The young man agreed. He came regularly and never missed a session. He was given respect and learned to respect others. By the end of the year he had the skills that would allow him to kill another human being. He also had the knowledge and wisdom of his teacher, which would ensure that he would only use his skills to help, never to hurt.

He learned to be a warrior, but a different kind of warrior from the kind he expected to be when he came in wanting to learn to kill. His belief, like so many young men today, had been "I better hurt you before you hurt me. If I've got to kill you, well that's just too bad." Without the guidance of an adult elder, he would never have learned that there was another warrior tradition.

I have found that teaching young men to deal with their anger and aggression helps me deal with my own. Helping them bring peace to their own lives helps me bring peace to my heart.

ACTION OPTION

Bring More Peace into Your World

Seek out a man you trust and talk to him about ways in which we might bring more peace to our neighborhoods, cities, and world. Talk to him about the school killings that are often in the news. Discuss the settings in your own community where you see the potential for violence. Think about things that you might do to make your world a more peaceful one in which to live.

The Role of Spirit Guide

Regardless of whether we have had positive, negative, or no experiences with religion growing up, as male elders we begin to be drawn to the spiritual dimension of life. We want to understand why we are here on this planet. We want to know what our life calling is and if we are following it. We have a need to find out about the essence of love and whether we are expressing it in our lives. We long to understand the meaning of life and death and what we need to do with our lives before it is our time to pass on.

These concerns are at the core of the restlessness we experience at this time of life. We feel stifled by our present existence, as though we were confined in a prison cell. We feel we need to escape, but we rarely know what is driving us. Many of us turn to what is familiar and slip into old patterns from our past. We become attracted to younger women, mistakenly hoping it will fill the spiritual hunger that is driving us.

Many of us tell our wives at this stage, "I love you, but I'm not in love with you." What we often mean, without being consciously aware of it, is "I'm searching for a larger sense of love that transcends the personal." Too many of us leave our wives at this stage, thinking that we are being trapped by our marriage. The truth is that we are really looking for the answers to spiritual questions.

Others of us lose ourselves in our work. If we don't feel successful, we try even harder to succeed. If we have done well at our work, we look for a new enterprise in which we can lose ourselves. But a spiritual hunger wants to be satisfied in us, and we don't know where to begin to get that need satisfied.

I have found there are a number of ways to connect with the spiritual dimension of life. The most accessible way is to go out into nature. Unfortunately, for many of us going into nature has involved loading up our camper and driving to national parks to see the "natural wonders" of our country. What we see in the parks is a little bit of nature and a lot of things made by humans.

ACTION OPTION

Explore the Meaning of Your Spirituality

Go to a beautiful place where you enjoy being alone. Take a piece of paper and title it "My Spirituality." Write about what spirituality means in your own life. Is it just about going to church or synagogue, or does it have a broader meaning to you? Write about times you feel the most spiritual and about how you'd like to see spirituality express itself in your life in the future. Find a person you trust and share the thoughts and feelings that have emerged from your writing.

The Role of Male Mentor

Kevin had become restless. He was 45 years old and at the top of his profession as human relations director for a large pharmaceutical company. He traveled all over the world and enjoyed the prestige and monetary benefits that his position afforded him. But something was missing. "I felt like I wanted to give something back, but I wasn't sure what I had to give or who would want to get it," he told me. He decided to cut back on his busy work schedule and see if he could understand what was next in his life.

Someone told him about the Big Brother/Big Sister program. He decided to try it and found it fulfilled a deep need that had opened up in him. "Since I became a 'big brother' to a teenage boy, my whole life seems to have grown larger," says Kevin. "In the past, my main satisfactions came from supporting my family and engineering business takeovers. It's kind of strange . . ." Kevin hesitated, looking for the right words. "But I feel a new kind of satisfaction from being a mentor to a young man. In my younger years, my body seemed to want sex and success. Now it seems to want to nurture, protect, and teach."

Mentoring is not only important for young men, but also for men who are in their 20s and 30s. One of the most important functions an elder can offer is teaching younger men how to be caring, responsible, open, and intimate husbands and fathers. Whether we have been successful in love and marriage, we have learned some important lessons. This is wisdom that young husbands and fathers need to receive from us.

Malidoma Somé is a wise elder I have known for some time. He was born in western Africa and initiated in the ancestral traditions of his tribe as a medicine man and diviner. He also holds three master's degrees, as well as two Ph.D.'s from the Sorbonne and Brandeis University. Since coming to the United States, he has been teaching the importance of these ancient roles to our modern society.

"Elders and mentors have an irreplaceable function in the life of any community," says Somé. "Without them, the young are lost—their overflowing energies wasted in useless pursuits. The old must live in the young like a grounding force that tames the tendency towards bold but senseless actions and shows them the path of wisdom. In the absence of elders, the impetuosity of youth becomes the slow death of the community."

ACTION OPTION

Honor Your Mentors

Write about the experiences you had with mentors growing up. Pay particular attention to those men who made a difference in your life. What did they do or say that made you feel valued and cared for? If there was no one who gave you that support, write about the ways this lack of mentoring influenced your life. Find a way to become a mentor to someone in your community who could benefit from the caring involvement of an older man.

Not only are these roles important to the well-being of the younger man and the community, they are critical to the well-being of the older man as well. One of the primary things that keep us alive and vital throughout our lives is the feeling that we are needed and have something important to contribute to the world. Finding ways to express the roles of peacemaker, spirit guide, and elder allows us to continue to grow.

If we do not find ways of expressing ourselves as elders we will regress to becoming adult-children. We become perpetual Peter Pans, afraid to grow up and take on the responsibilities and pleasures of elderhood. If we don't engage this stage in a positive way, we begin to stagnate and go downhill—physically, emotionally, and spiritually.

This is why we see so many men in their middle years, between 40 and 55, acting like adult-children. Some of them become sick and need to be taken care of like a child. Others perpetually search for the latest gadgets and toys and a young beauty to fulfill all their wants and wishes like a spoiled child at Christmas. What they need is to find a way to give to others. They need to feel they are needed and have something significant to offer their families, their communities, and their world.

The Reemergence of the Lost Fathers

The 20th century was not a good time for the relationship between fathers and their children. As we have felt more disconnected from our work, we feel less passion and purpose in our lives. One of the ways this loss expresses itself is when we feel we have less to offer our children. It's not just that our monetary contribution has become more and more uncertain, but with it our feeling of worth and value in all areas of our lives.

But this is changing. Fathers are silent no longer. More and more are speaking out, reclaiming their place with their children. We see this trend in a number of major men's movements going on throughout the country and around the world. There is a great deal of diversity: from the Mankind Project and the Sterling men's organization to the born-again Christian Promise Keepers and the African American Million Man Marchers, from organizations that have a feminist approach and are fighting for more rights for women to men's rights organizations that are concerned with keeping men connected with their families.

There is a growing recognition of the importance of men in their families while the children are small, as well as after they grow up. One of the leaders of this movement is Warren Farrell, who has been researching and writing about men's and women's issues for over 30 years. In his most recent book, *Father and Child Reunion,* Farrell offers compelling evidence that supports the unique value that men have in the lives of their families. Fatherhood has a wonderful spiritual value for every member of the family.

ACTION OPTION

Seek Out Your Children and Parents

If you have children, go see each one and talk about the kind of fathering they received from you when they were growing up. Find out what they need now. You may find that you were a better father than you thought and that your children still need you even after they are grown. If you don't have children, go talk to your parents or other older adults who had an influence on your life and tell them how their support affected you.

New Roles for New Men

Nurturing the Spirit of Children

Most of us love babies, but we usually don't develop the same degree of body connection that a woman has. We don't carry a baby in our body and we don't breast-feed. As a result we never know the spiritual bond that is possible between an adult and an infant.

I had occasion to get a tiny glimpse into that experience when my daughter gave birth to my granddaughter. Her labor was long and intense, but we were able to leave the hospital the next morning. My wife and I drove our daughter and her new baby to their apartment. We had gotten a motel room and planned to spend a week to help them get settled.

By nighttime my wife and daughter were both exhausted. I agreed to stay with my daughter and the baby while my wife returned to our hotel room. It was wonderful and very moving to hold a newborn baby as she experienced her first day of life in the world. Since my daughter needed to rest, I offered to keep my granddaughter with me. I said I'd call her if I needed help.

I lay down on the couch with my granddaughter snuggled up to my bare chest. As she began to suck on my shoulder, I was given the gift of feeling a small part of what a mother experiences. It felt like the most natural thing in the world. I felt a connection to the spirit of life that I had never experienced before.

When my own children were born, I held them close. But in the intimacy of our bed, my wife held the babies close to her body and I surrounded them both with my arms. Holding my granddaughter was a different experience. The bond was so strong and the feeling of love so great, I wept with joy.

I knew if guys could experience just one night with their children in this way, it would make all the difference in the world. Dads would not want to leave their children and would do more to keep relationships healthy and intact. The world would be a better place, and the spirit of what poet Robert Bly called "male mothers" would enhance the lives of men, women, and children.

Honoring the Spirit of Life's Passing

When Carlin's mother came to live with us during the last months of her life, I was uneasy at first. I wasn't sure how it would be to take care of someone who didn't have long to spend on earth. I agreed out of a sense of duty and a desire to give my wife the support she needed to take care of her mother.

I was not prepared for the spiritual gift I received. In the first days and weeks of her time with us, I would talk to her and hold her hand. I told her how glad I was that she could be with us and that we could make this time as comfortable for her as possible. What began as my trying to say the words that I thought she'd want to hear quickly became real.

Taking care of someone who is dying was not at all like I expected it would be. Rather than being morbid and sad, I found that my heart opened up the more I was with her. There was a peacefulness and calm that spread throughout our house. Since my wife was a hospice volunteer she knew how to take care of her mom, and we were supported by doctors and nurses who gave us the medications that would keep her from experiencing pain.

In the last days I was able to sit with her a lot. She didn't talk and just looked into my eyes. Looking back at her, I felt like I was looking into the face of God. There was so much love and acceptance that I knew I need never fear death or worry about how I would leave the world.

After having the experience with Carlin's mom, my life has been transformed. I found that being with someone as they make the transition from life to death is one of the most profound spiritual experiences we can have. I recommend that everyone seek out an opportunity to have such an experience.

Once we embrace the spiritual side of life we feel called upon to share our experiences with others. This is not through preaching or proselytizing, but simply by living in a way that is an expression of spirit. I feel bathed in the spiritual dimension when I visit Sidney, my teacher from graduate school, who is now in his late 80s. Any time I am with him, I feel special. I feel loved and cared for. It's as though the spirit of love comes through him. I also feel that I am in the presence of wisdom. He is always teaching little life lessons, all of which act to clear the curtain of fear and doubt from my eyes. I feel seen, heard, recognized, and appreciated.

It's as though I am in the presence of a man who is at peace with himself and the world, a being who is a conduit for all that is loving and beautiful in the world. I hope that I can learn to radiate that kind of spirit to others as I get older.

PART V

The Men Alive Program for Healthy Relationships

CHAPTER 13

Inside a Men's Support Group

> The grief in men has been increasing steadily since the start of the Industrial Revolution and the grief has reached a depth now that cannot be ignored.
>
> —Robert Bly

Becoming a Man among Men

It was 1975 and my first marriage was not going well. I was 32, we had been married nine years, and our two children were 6 and 3. For my wife, Candace, the women's liberation movement was in full swing. She was involved in the local women's center and had lots of friends and many projects she was deeply connected with.

I felt envious and left out. When my friend Brad said he was starting a men's group I was intrigued. However, I was also reluctant to get involved with a bunch of guys. What would we talk about? What would they want from me? I saw other men as competitors for job promotions or for women. How would I protect myself? What would I do if one of them was gay? Homophobia is strong among heterosexual guys. Though my rational mind accepts people being gay or straight, fears still run deep. I still had secret worries about my manhood and sexuality.

But on my friend's recommendation I joined. It was not like anything I could have imagined. Over the next months we talked about things I didn't think men talked about. We shared our fears of loss, our worries about being successful, our problems in our relationships with women.

We were a mixed group, single and married, in our 20s and 30s. There was a counselor, an artist, a potter, a contractor, a salesman, and a farmer. What we had in common was that we were all men in search of our foundations—the daimon, the true self, the inner voice that would direct our lives.

Confronting Jealousy

After meeting for about six months we had an encounter that changed the way we saw ourselves and each other. Gary was single and had fallen in love with Sue. He was enthralled and excited, as we all can be in the first bloom of love. As it turned out, Rod also had a crush on Sue since they'd first met in the first grade. There was clearly a good deal of tension between the two men that permeated the group. But no one knew what to say or how to deal with this triangle.

When we were at parties where we were all present and Sue was in attendance, she seemed to be interested in both men. I will never forget the group session in which Gary broke the silence. "Let's be honest," Gary said, looking directly at Rod. "I know you're interested in Sue." I remember tensing, feeling that this could turn violent. The only way I had ever experienced guys solving problems like these was with their fists.

To my surprise, violence didn't break out, but more words were spoken. Slow and halting, but direct and honest. Gary continued. "And I know . . . as sure as I'm sitting here . . . that regardless of our friendship . . . that if there was a choice between keeping our friendship and you getting a shot at Sue . . . you'd choose her."

I thought, "Hell yes, that's just the way it is in the world. Guys are friends only as long as there's no competition for a job or a woman. When it gets down to it, each of us is on his own." But Rod had a different reality. "Before the group, or even a few months in, you'd probably be right," he answered in his slow, rich southern accent. "But now that we've gotten to be friends and we've developed a bond as a group, things have changed." In a voice that had more emotion than the usually quiet Rod had let us see he continued: "The truth is that our friendship means more to me than having Sue or any woman." We couldn't believe what we were hearing. Could this really be happening? Could friendship between men be as important as Rod was saying it was? "If you tell me Sue is important to you, I'll back away." Rod's words and his manner, the calm and clear way he voiced them, left no doubt that he was serious.

When, over the next weeks and months, we saw his behavior match the words, we realized we had entered a new era in our group experience and were opening up new ways that men could truly trust each other. We began to support each other in traditional and not-so-traditional ways.

We helped each other move, did projects on each others' houses, lent each other money (and paid it back when we said we would), planned parties together, and played music. But we also listened to each other when we were feeling down and confused. We offered advice when asked, not when our egos needed to make a point. We hugged when we were happy and received comforting when we were sad. We even nursed one another when we were sick.

The Gift of a Nurturing Man

I remember the absolute gift and wonder of having a male friend nurture and care for me when I couldn't care for myself. I had a high fever and a flu that had lasted for three or four days. I felt miserable and alone. My wife and I had separated two months previously, and I had been living in a friend's converted garage while she remained with the kids in what had always been our house, but was mine no longer.

One of the truths I had learned over the years is that when you're sick, you need a woman to take care of you. If I needed help, I had to get it from a woman. It wasn't even anything I questioned. Just as a baby goes to his mother when he needs to nurse, a man goes to a woman when he needs care and nurture. Men don't nurse babies, and men don't take care of other men when we're sick.

I thought of every woman friend I knew. I called a few and none were home. I even thought about calling my soon-to-be ex-wife. I knew any care she would bring would be mixed with anger and blame. As sick as I was, I thought I'd even accept that if I could have a woman come and take care of me.

Before I could call her, the phone rang. It was Steve, one of the men in the group. He asked me how things were going, and I immediately shifted into my "guy" way of responding. "I'm OK," I said before I could even think about whether I could tell him the truth about how miserable I was.

Instead of responding in kind, with a quick "Well, OK, I'll catch you later, see you at group," he listened to my feelings, not my words. "You sound sick," Steve said directly but kindly. "How are you *really* feeling?" His response floored me. I nearly broke into tears. I admitted that I felt terrible, hadn't been able to keep any food down, and had been lying on my living room couch for days watching television and trying to ignore my illness.

"I'll be right over," he said. And, to my utter surprise, I actually got a knock at my door. He came with some groceries and started to make me some chicken soup, which we both laughed at. "Yeah, well, pretend it's like your mother used to make you," he said. I told him I didn't need to pretend. My mother was a lousy cook and Campbell's was one of her mainstay meals. After eating a little, I felt better, as much from the friendship as from the food.

Confronting Homophobia

After we talked awhile, he asked if I wanted a massage. I thought, "I'd love one." But right after that I felt a wave of fear. "I know Steve's not gay, but why would he want to give a man a massage? What would he think if I accepted? What if I liked it; would he think *I* was gay?" All this went through my head in a few brief seconds.

I was beginning to see how much my fear of homosexuality had limited my ability to experience my full potential as a man. I had flashes of memory from my childhood. I remembered being ridiculed as a sissy, a pansy, or a fag if I wouldn't fight. Showing sadness or allowing oneself to cry was seen as unmanly. If you weren't manly in the traditional sense of being tough, unfeeling, and uncaring, you were suspected of being gay.

It's tragic the way our culture has taken the soft, gentle, and nurturing aspects of our manhood and made these qualities acceptable only in women and gay men, and then made being gay a horrible thing. As an adult I came to realize that I didn't have to be tough; I could be gentle. I didn't have to be unfeeling; I could express a range of emotions. I didn't have to be uncaring; I could care about other people, even men. I learned that being gay or straight has nothing to do with being manly. If you're a man, everything you do is manly.

Even so, homophobia dies slowly. I still had a moment of hesitation before I gratefully accepted Steve's offer of a massage. I stretched out on the couch, and he massaged my back, my neck, and my shoulders. It felt wonderful. I felt cared for and nurtured in a way that I thought was not possible to receive from a man. I realized how limiting was my belief that nurturing and care can only come from a woman.

The Safety of a Mature Men's Group

When I moved out of the area I joined another group, which seemed to begin where my other one left off. Like me, many of the men had been in groups before. We were older and ranged in age from our early 30s to early 50s. We've now been together going on 22 years.

We would start each group session with a check-in. It was a chance to open up to each other and tell the truth about what was really going on in our lives. We were able to talk about the hopes and the frustrations we were experiencing in our relationships with the women in our lives. One of the men who was gay talked about similar experiences. But he also talked about additional stresses.

Since he worked for a large pharmaceutical company, he felt he had to keep his relationships totally private. "It makes me angry," he told us, "that I have to worry about what I say when my friend calls me at work." The pressures weren't just at work: "When we go out, I have to worry that someone might see us and guess that we are more than good friends."

It was nice to have a safe place to talk about our anger, fear, and sadness. One of the men suffered from lifelong depression and had never told anyone how difficult it was just to get through the day. "It's like living in a black cloud," he said. "I am surrounded by darkness and I don't know whether I will ever see the light."

Another man talked about the shame he experienced while growing up with an alcoholic mother. I shared my early memories of my father's mood swings and suicide attempts. Together we began to see what it meant to be men. We had all grown up in a time when keeping your problems to yourself was the norm.

At first it was difficult to open up, but over time it got easier and easier. In fact, it became the highlight of my week. No matter how difficult things were at work or how stressful life was at home with the family, the men's group was a refuge where I could just be myself and not feel like I had to take care of others.

Getting Naked Together

In addition to getting to know each other and having a place we could be ourselves, we devised various exercises to help expand our awareness and learn more about what it meant to be a man.

One of the most memorable for me was the time we got naked together. Growing up, the only time I ever took my clothes off around other guys was in the locker room. Those experiences were often shameful. As was the case with a lot of boys who were different (I was short and developed early), the locker room was a place where I was teased mercilessly. According to the bigger boys who ruled the locker room, there was always something wrong with my body.

Now I was grown and with a group of guys I had come to trust. The exercise was that each of us would take our clothes off and stand in front of the other men. We would then get feedback about our bodies, but it would be feedback of a new kind. We would be told what the other men liked about our bodies. I remember feeling increasingly anxious as my turn approached.

I always felt too short and wished I was taller. I felt my thighs were too heavy and that my nose was too long. The old locker room fears began to come back. By the time I was standing in front of the men I was sweating and worrying about sweating. The responses I received were so healing I can still remember them 20 years later.

Everything I heard was positive. The men liked the color of my eyes, the pattern of the hair on my chest, the muscles in my calves. They saw things from a uniquely male perspective, and their validation helped me validate myself in a way that no woman ever could. It was as though a loving father and a group of loving uncles all told you how unique and perfect you were.

I had thought that only women had problems with body image. It wasn't until I had the experience of standing in front of other men that all the memories of shame I felt growing up began to emerge. Just as much of the shame had come from being judged by other boys in my youth, the healing validation I received from these men replaced the shame with acceptance and pride. After that I was a lot more comfortable in my body.

A Group That Can Last Forever

We've experienced divorces, marriages, 50th wedding anniversaries, the death of a loved dog, the birth of a man's first child, job promotions and firings, the loss when two men moved away, the excitement and fear when two new men were added (the newest man came into the group 14 years ago), business successes and failures, problems with teenage children and problems with adult children who still act like teenagers, health problems with our wives, the joys and strains of one man's retirement, the death of parents, and a man diagnosed and treated for prostate cancer.

We have committed to being together for the rest of our lives and drinking a toast to each man when he dies. We have a contest to see who will die last. The last one to make it to heaven (if there is such a place, we figure we'll have to go there, since at least one of us is heaven material and they can't split up the group) has to buy beers, in perpetuity, for the rest of the guys.

Two years ago we celebrated being together for 20 years by chartering a yacht and spending a week in Alaska. Planning the trip was a trip in itself. It took us nearly 3 years to agree on a place all seven of us wanted to go to. One reason why it may have taken so long was that we liked to discuss the trip at wonderful dinners complemented by superb wine. One of our members owns a vineyard in the Napa Valley. Although we all had different ideas, there were some things we agreed upon.

We wanted to go somewhere that would be memorable. Given our ages and temperaments, we were looking for a place that was simple yet luxurious, wild yet comfortable, magnificent yet easy to get to, close to water yet with access to wonderful experiences on the land. We also had to come up with something we all could afford, even with saving our money for three years. Alaska seemed to meet our requirements.

It met and exceeded them. We motored through some of the most beautiful scenery in the world and fished for salmon and halibut, crabs and clams. We ate what we caught and went back for more. We walked on glaciers and got close enough to bears to feel the power of their presence. We watched eagles soar and orcas sound.

We celebrated our time together, talked about the past, and thought about the future. We wondered what we'd do at our next 20-year celebration. Our eldest member would be 90 and our youngest would be 68. One or more of us could be dead, and it wouldn't necessarily be the oldest of us. You never knew.

There were some things we did know for certain. We would be together in 20 years. We would mark it with a celebration. Though we often experienced disagreements, some of them quite serious, we would still be friends. We will still be learning new things, learning more about what it means to be a man and what we could pass on to younger men.

Initiation: Learning What It Means to Be a Male Elder

Our men's group had been together nearly 15 years when we decided something was missing in our lives. As we approached and moved into middle age, we found we were wrestling with similar questions.

- What have I done with my life?
- When I die, will I be remembered?
- Have I made a difference in the world?
- What do I have to teach the younger generation?

- How do I relate to a partner who is getting older?
- What do I do about my flagging sexual desire?
- What do I do when my sexual desire is there but my body won't perform?
- How do I deal with my own aging?

Between ourselves we weren't able to come up with answers that satisfied us. We felt we needed something more.

The opportunity came in the form of a men's weekend sponsored by the Mankind Project. We were drawn by the double-edged goals of the weekend, which were (1) to initiate men into a mature masculinity, to lead lives of integrity, connection to feeling, and a renewed responsibility for their personal mission in the world, and (2) to be of service to the community.

The group flew down to San Diego, then drove 2 hours toward Mount Palomar. It was clear we were entering a very different world. The landscape was magnificent—the view from the top made me think I was halfway to heaven—but what went on in the 48 hours we spent there was as spectacular as the view. In a notebook I kept, shortly after we returned, I wrote, "The weekend was transformative, for us as a group and for each of us individually. It was a true initiation, a rite of passage, a celebration of manhood, and an opportunity to fully develop our life-purpose."

Although it all seemed mysterious while we were going through it, looking back on the weekend I can see that there were three stages typical of initiations that have been held in tribal cultures for thousands of years. There was a *descent,* where we left our traditional nine-to-five existence and entered a new world of the initiate. There was an *ordeal,* where we each faced our own demons that had limited our lives and kept us cut off from ourselves and those we loved. Finally, there was a *homecoming,* where we joined together to consolidate our new learnings and to integrate them into our lives back home.

Awakening the Masculine Soul

Each of us came out with a clearer sense of our calling and what we had to offer each other and our community. In my experience I was here to help men get in touch with their deepest longings. The phrase that captured it for me was "help men awaken their masculine soul." Later I refined it to "helping men live long and well." Returning from the weekend, I felt I had a clear sense of where I was going and what my unique contribution was in the larger scheme of things.

Just as adolescence is a time for initiation that can help a boy become a man, so, too, is middlescence a period that can help a man move from the first half of life to the second. The Swiss psychoanalyst Carl Jung described the journey we must all make, if we are fortunate to have made it this far: "Wholly unprepared, we embark upon the second half of life. . . . we take the step into the afternoon of life; worse still we take this step with the false assumption that our truths and ideals will serve as before. But we cannot live the afternoon of life according to the program of life's morning—for what was great in the morning will be little at evening, and what in the morning was true will at evening have become a lie."

Seeing men in the second half of our lives desperately holding on to the glories of our youth is like watching animals in the zoo. There is a compulsive restlessness about our behavior. We go back and forth from one side of our cage to the other, anxious and at the same time bored. I believe what we are looking for at this stage of life is to discover what things we need to let go of from the morning of our lives. We also need to discover what we will need for the evening of our lives that we have not yet developed.

I believe that joining a men's group is one of the most vital and important things we can do to ensure that we make it through the evening of our lives with passion, purpose, and the gift of giving. "I don't know what your destiny will be," said Albert Schweitzer, who spent 50 years of his life serving his fellow man in the oppressive heat of the African jungle, "but one thing I do know; the only ones among you who will be really happy are those who have sought and found how to serve."

A Modern-Day Vision Quest: Gregory's Story

After being together for over 20 years, the trust level in the group was considerable. Each of us found that as we approached and moved through midlife there were certain barriers that we faced. The group provided the support to help us break through the constraints that kept us from being able to find our true selves.

Gregory found himself in a rut. On the surface, his life was successful. His relationship with his wife was flourishing. He had reached a point in his business where things were going smoothly. However, he seemed to have lost touch with his larger vision, his spiritual longings, and the deep wellsprings of his deeper passions.

We had developed a process for helping us break out of our old patterns. If a man asked for help the rest of the group gathered without him and came up with a collective plan. The agreement was that if we asked for help we would do whatever the group felt was best for us.

For all of us that was a huge leap of faith. We had been brought up with various degrees of distrust of other men. As adults we had learned to keep our cards close to our chests. We rarely let another man know that we were hurting or stuck, and we never let another man have control over our lives.

Yet each of us had gone through the process. Here's Gregory's story.

> After thinking about it for a long while, I finally put my fears aside and got up the courage to ask the other men for help. As I knew they would, the group asked me to leave. They said they would call me when it was time for me to come back.
>
> I remember walking around for what seemed like many hours. I was very anxious. I didn't have a clue about what the group would suggest. Questions ran through my mind. Would they want me to do something that I felt I wouldn't be able to do? Would my wife go along with some major change that might affect her life? Could they really come up with something that would help me find my path at this time of my life?
>
> I also felt grateful that the group would spend hours working out a plan that would help me. I looked forward to their support with a mixture of excitement and anxiety. When I returned the group had decided that what I really needed was a modern-day vision quest. I knew that Native Americans spent time alone for many days without eating or drinking, seeking visions that would guide their future. Is this what they had in mind for me?
>
> Since I am an educator and *theoretically* have a summer off where I don't work, the group decided to take over the direction of that time. The goal was for me to spend a lot of time *by* myself and *for* myself. They told me that I had spent the first part of my life very much oriented towards pleasing others.
>
> In order to move into the next phase of my life, I would need to change my focus. I needed time to go inside myself and consider who I am and where I am going. There were some interesting restrictions that they placed on my activities throughout the summer. They didn't want me to indulge in entertainments and diversions like movies or books. I was told not to use any mind-altering substances, including alcohol.
>
> My time began with a camping trip by myself high in the Sierra Nevada range of northern California. I spent four days

alone with myself. I had to confront a lot of trust issues. Would the men really follow through and do what they said? Would they really handle me with the love and care I needed?

I was at an elevation of 10,000 feet, and it was crystal clear and very cold at night. There was a brilliant full moon during that period. It was exquisitely pristine and difficult. Each day I hiked up into the granite mountains that surrounded my camp. The stark clarity of the place enabled me to think deeply about my own life. Each day I wrote in my journal. Questions surfaced from deep inside me. Where was I going? What were my real gifts? Could I make a difference in my own small way?

The next part of the journey involved a seven-day workshop on basic trust that I attended with my wife, Andrea. It was a very emotional week. The experience brought us closer together.

I next spent five days in San Francisco. It was a kind of urban retreat, in some ways quite similar to what I had experienced in the mountains. I did a lot of meditating and hiking. In was fun and interesting to pretend that San Francisco was nothing more than a populated Sierra Nevada, and I would just hike through it. I remember hiking down Market Street, observing the fauna and flora of the place. It gave me a whole new perspective on my life in the city.

The final week was spent at a Catholic monastery. The priests there allowed people to come for times of contemplation and meditation. I had some real misgivings about coming because I still have a lot of anger toward the Catholic Church, which goes back to childhood experiences.

Although I had planned to stay by myself and avoid interacting with the priests who lived there, that didn't happen. I was drawn to one of the priests and ended up having a number of great conversations with him. It was just the right thing that I carried my anger to him because he was extremely understanding and sensitive. I was able to release a lot of the old anger that I had carried all this time. I was also able to cry.

A lot of blocks were freed up. As I left the monastery I felt I had left some of the hurts and anger from my past. I returned to the day-to-day world with a new perspective on my life and future directions.

Before the summer retreat I don't think I would have had the courage and the vision to do what I had to do to make it work.

All in all, I couldn't have felt more blessed to be around a group of men that cared this much about me. My life is much better and significantly deeper as a result. The summer experience

> would not have happened without the support of these men. I feel infinitely richer as a result.

The group was also blessed to be able to guide Gregory and help create an experience that was so rich and fruitful. In the 22 years we have been together I have been amazed at what we are able to create together. Individually we can go only so far. As a group we can achieve things we never thought were possible.

I can't think of any better way to help you move ahead on your journey into the second half of life than to join a men's group.

My first group was started by one guy who saw the value and invited a few friends to join him. It grew from there. The same thing can happen with you.

The Importance of Men's Groups

In our modern world, men's groups have come to be laughed at. The image often portrayed by the media is that of a bunch of guys running around the woods trying to get in touch with the wild man within. This type of ridicule seems to occur whenever men and women try to break out of the old sexist roles that have kept us locked up. When women began to change in the 1960s, they were portrayed as bra-burning bitches.

Men's groups and lodges have been around for a long time, and their importance was once more fully recognized than it has recently. Psychologist Tom Daly describes the evolution of men's fraternal organizations: "The desire for knowledge of the mysteries of manhood has spawned men's lodges and groups throughout human history. In the recent past, in the mid-to-late 1800's, there was a huge stirring among men that spawned the Elks, Moose, Lions, Rotarians, Kiwanis, Optimists, and other fraternal service organizations that are part of our current social fabric."

The hunger that drives us toward gender-specific groups is the same now as it was in the 1800s and throughout the long span of human history. Chris Harding, a men's movement leader, recognizes the similarity of needs that spawned the traditional men's lodges and modern men's groups.

> Though there are profound differences between men's groups of today and yesteryear, there are surprisingly many parallels. To name just four:

1. Exploration of ways to fulfill spiritual needs not adequately met by organized religion
2. Abiding, unquenchable thirst for initiation
3. Search for father figures and role models
4. The need for a safe space in which to shed everyday persona.

ACTION OPTION

Learn about Men's Groups

Read a book on men's groups. Seek out and talk to a man who is a member of a men's group. Join a men's group or start your own.

I can tell you that being a part of a men's group has been, and continues to be, one of the most valuable experiences I've had in my life. We live in a stressful world, and all indications are that the stress levels will increase along with world population, increasing the consumption of our resources and the resulting pollution. Further, we live in a society that is becoming more fragmented and violent. For me, being part of a men's group is as essential as eating well, getting enough exercise, keeping my hormones in balance, and following all the other health measures I have recommended. Don't leave out this vital part of a complete health regimen.

CHAPTER 14

Gender Shifting and Male Magnetism in the Second Half of Life

> Don't be the man you're supposed to be; be the father you would like to have had.
>
> —Letty Pogebrin

JUST WHEN I THOUGHT I'd finally gotten comfortable with what it means to be a man and what a woman really wants, the ground beneath me began to shift and I was thrown off balance. Carlin and I had been married 10 years and had settled into a nice routine. I had the major moneymaking role with a career that often took me on the road.

Carlin's career brought in less money and allowed her to spend time at home with the children. Although our marriage was far from being a traditional one like that of our parents, it was stable and satisfying. We were both making our way through the menopause passage.

After recovering from surgery when I had an adrenal tumor removed, I decided that I wanted to relax more and work less. We moved to the country and, to my surprise, I loved the slower pace. I could spend hours splitting wood and prided myself on spending quality time in the hammock each day. Where in the past I loved to travel, now I had no interest in exotic places. I just wanted to stay at home.

Carlin, on the other hand, began to expand her work. She found she was becoming increasingly sought after as a counselor and spiritual mentor. She began to travel more and deepened her work with women. Even her time at home was much more demanding. She planted a city-block-sized garden and became a farmer with tasks that needed to be accomplished each day and throughout the seasons. She watered, fertilized, weeded, planted, and harvested. She terraced the hillside and pounded in iron rebar to shore up the boards that held her fruit trees. She put in an irrigation system that had to be monitored and cleaned periodically.

She was so busy that I had to remind her that we needed to take time for us. That used to be her role. Now it was me who was suggesting a day to ourselves. It seemed to be my turn to read relationship articles and books to get clues about keeping our marriage alive and well. We seemed nearly to have reversed roles.

Gender Shifting: A New Stage of Life

I found a similar pattern with friends and clients. Many couples become confused, and even frightened, over this shift in behavior. We long for the past when things seemed, if not more comfortable, at least more predictable. We become confused and despondent. We don't understand what's going on. Often we blame each other or blame ourselves. It's not uncommon for one member of the couple to have an affair during this stage of life.

This change is particularly difficult for us men. We have spent a lifetime building a sense of male identity based on certain "manly" behaviors. Now we don't have interest or energy for the old practices. Are we losing our manhood, becoming more like a woman? This thought is terrifying to most of us.

It's difficult for us to realize that this gender shift does not mean that a guy is losing his manhood. In fact, it means his manhood is expanding. I still remember the opening scenes of *The Godfather,* in which we see Marlon Brando at the wedding of his daughter. He has a gentleness about him. He bestows blessings on the younger men and women and shares his wisdom and life experience. Although he doesn't show the fire and aggression of a young man, no one doubts his masculinity. One of the last scenes in the movie shows Brando in his garden tending his flowers. Clearly a new aspect of masculinity has been developing and finds its full expression in the later years of life.

The Three Stages of Life: Prereproductive, Reproductive, Postreproductive

In the prereproductive years before adolescence, males and females are more alike than different. There is an integration between the outgoing, assertive sides of ourselves and the gentler, emotional sides. We played together without shame. There was a group of us who would play house together (mostly girls, but a few boys) some days, then on other days we would play baseball (mostly boys, but a few girls).

I remember being around 10 years old and feeling such love and affection for my buddies. We loved sports, but we also loved music. I still remember, as though it was yesterday, the evening Jack called me on the phone. We still had those big, black stand-up phones with the large, heavy earpiece.

He was so excited to play me a new song he had just gotten. He sang along as he played the record for me. We both loved it. It spoke so truly to our friendship and to our time of life. There was no conflict between being a rough-and-ready guy and a guy who could put his arms around his buddy and sing his praises. It was a time we wished would last forever.

But then came puberty with all its hormonal, physical, emotional, and sexual changes. Up until then, our boy friends and girl friends seemed much more similar than different. Now the differences began to be apparent as the dating and mating dance began to take over our lives.

Later in the adult years our initial desire for sex often turns into a desire to have a family. During the child-rearing years men and women continue to be different. The battle of the sexes is in full swing at the same time we are trying to learn to live together and raise a family.

In the third age of life, during the postreproductive years, men and women have an opportunity to experience a part of the adult life cycle that had been sacrificed during the reproductive years. During the reproductive years a man needed to suppress a lot of his nurturing, caring aspects. Think of a man who did not want to leave his wife and children to go hunting because he was so emotionally connected it tore him up to leave. For the good of his family he submerged those parts of himself. Think of a woman who didn't want to stay at home to nurture her small children because the call of the wild was such a strong pull that she needed to follow it. She suppressed the wild woman in her for the good of the family.

One of the critical differences between males and females at this stage of life is that menopause heralds the end of the reproductive years for women, while andropause brings about a profound change for men yet still allows them reproductive choice. Since men *can* reproduce more children there is often an urge to seek out younger women who are still in the reproductive years. This is the source of a great deal of conflict between men and women.

However, many of us are quite content to leave our reproductive life behind along with the desire to search out and bed as many young, attractive women as we can find. We want to deepen our relationship with our mate and to allow ourselves to experience the joys of an expanded masculinity in the second half of life.

Other men are not ready to move on to the third phase of life. They like the feeling of perpetual youth. These are the men who have trouble feeling sexual desire for their older mates. They are the ones who think the number and strength of their erections is the mark of their manhood. There is nothing wrong with these desires, even though older women may not like them because they are afraid they signal that a man no longer finds them attractive and is ready to leave. Ultimately a man needs to decide for himself when he is ready to move on to the third phase.

In the third phase of life we can reclaim the parts of ourselves we had to give up during the reproductive years. We can take back the feelings and behaviors we had turned over to women, and women can assert the parts of themselves they have had to keep hidden. We are not so driven by the reproductive desires. We can become less driven and competitive, more comfortable with ourselves and others.

Gender Crossing: Becoming All That You Can Be

For years, when my wife, Carlin, and I went out together, I was the one who drove while she sat in the passenger seat. It never occurred to us to do otherwise. We'd leave the house together and she'd automatically go to the right side of the car while I would move toward the left. I'd get in behind the wheel and she'd get in behind the glove compartment.

She'd sometimes offer to drive when I seemed tired or we were on a long trip together. "I'm fine. No problem," I'd answer, and continue to drive on. Even when I'd be dead tired, I would pull off the road and take a few winks of sleep before driving on. There was no logical reason why Carlin shouldn't have driven. She was an excellent driver, but it just didn't feel right.

Something strange began to happen somewhere around my 40th birthday. Occasionally I would "let" her drive when she asked. As time went on, I even asked her if she'd like to drive. Later, I'd actually ask her if she would drive. Somewhere along the line I found that I was heading for the glove compartment side of the car and Carlin was getting in behind the wheel.

I found I was enjoying letting go of the role of being in charge and always having to know where I was going, even when I was lost. I liked being able to relax, look out the window, and enjoy the scenery. I began to see things on regular drives that I had never noticed before when I was concentrating on the road ahead and watching for danger.

I remembered my father always telling me that the way to avoid an accident was always to be looking three or four cars ahead as well as at the cars immediately in front and behind. I'd spent my adult life on the road constantly looking for danger. It felt so good to take a break from that.

I also found, to my surprise, that Carlin liked driving. She genuinely enjoyed the feel of the car and the experience of navigating through traffic. For her 50th birthday I enrolled her in the world-famous Bondurant racing-school program. It has a special program for teaching highway safety skills and high-performance driving. She learned to get her car out of a skid, how to handle a car safely at high speeds, and how to think like a racecar driver. She said it was the best birthday present she had ever gotten.

I remember the weekend she was at the driving school. I spent the day relaxing at home, tending the garden, enjoying the summer sunshine, and talking to our grandchildren on the phone. It was a strange feeling. I kept thinking, "It should be me at the driving school. What will our friends think when I tell them my wife is off circling a racetrack?" I imagined them thinking, "Well, we know who wears the pants in *that* family."

But beyond the fears of losing face with my friends was the deeper reality that I was definitely doing what I wanted to do and that Carlin was doing what she wanted to do. I know I didn't feel unmanly. I felt proud that my wife wanted to drive well and that she had the guts to attend that kind of high-powered school. I felt safer driving with her knowing there was a highly trained driver at the wheel. Most of all I liked the luxury of slowing my own life down, taking time to enjoy nature and nurture my children and grandchildren.

I felt like there was a whole side of me that was now beginning to grow and develop. In my earlier years I knew I was successful in the outer world, but often felt scared and unsure of myself in the inner world. I always had to have something going. Being alone with myself bordered on the terrifying. Sitting still was a torture.

I felt like I was a tree that been standing a long time, but with roots that barely held it up. Now I was extending my roots deep into the earth. I didn't have to keep striving to go higher. Now I could begin going deeper. I didn't have to spend all my days and nights planning how I could move up in the world. I could quietly put my energy into learning how to extend myself more broadly out into my community.

In my earlier years I wanted more than anything to be successful in my life. But I realized that success had more to do with personal achievement than it had to do with giving back to the community. I also came to see that personal success was very much tied to the wounds I experienced in childhood. I wanted to be financially successful so that women would be attracted to me and respect me. I wanted stable employment so that women wouldn't talk to me like I remembered my mother and her friends talking about their husbands—with pity and disdain.

I realized that I had been driven toward success by my childhood fears. I wanted to prove to my mother that I was the kind of man she could admire. I had tried to prove to every woman that I met that I would never be weak, I would never lose face, I would never fail. It was a losing battle. It's why so many men become depressed at this time of life. We are in the last stages of a war within ourselves that can never be won. We must either move beyond the battlefield or we will die.

I finally understood what Albert Einstein meant when, in his later years, he advised, "Try not to become a man of success, rather become a man of value." He recognized that success in some ways is illusory, based upon following someone else's dream. It is one-dimensional and self-centered. Becoming a man of value implies something much larger and deeper. It involves new kinds of relationships with our loved ones and with others in the world outside our families.

Resisting the Shame of Becoming a "Magnetic" Man

In the second half of life men seem to be drawn back toward home, back toward the center. We are drawn by what anthropologist Angeles Arrien calls the "magnetic" dimension of life. This dimension of life is involved with the inner world, with self-reflection, family connections, and intimacy. Women are driven by the opposite, what Arrien calls the "dynamic" dimension. The adventurer in them begins to assert itself and they want to move outward toward the periphery.

However, we live in a society that values the dynamic dimension much more than the magnetic. Women who embrace the dynamic aspects of themselves, though it may cause discomfort for those they are close to, are generally respected. On the other hand, men who embrace the magnetic aspects of life are often shamed.

This is frequently added to the shame we feel about ourselves from earlier periods of our lives. During the reproductive years we are often shamed for being away from home too much, always working, never emotionally available to our wives and children. Now, in the second half of life, we are often shamed for being at home too much and our lack of interest in going out as much as we once did. "He just wants to sit around the house. He never wants to *do* anything." This is a lament I hear from many midlife women.

The shame becomes a disease that destroys a man's sense of self-worth as it destroys the love, trust, and respect that is necessary for men and women to move successfully through the andropause passage. However, if we understand the natural rhythms of male and female maturity, we will understand that this gender shift is necessary and desirable in a relationship.

Magnetic Sex: Slow Hands and an Easy Touch

Since Carlin and I have been going through menopause and andropause, our sexual desires have shifted. There was a time when she was much less interested in sex. I equated sex with having intercourse or at least some kind of "penis play" resulting in orgasm. She would want more romance, touching, playing, and fun. Sometimes that's all she seemed to want. I would tell her that I'd be more romantic if she would be more interested in having sex. She'd tell me that she would be more interested in having sex if we spent more time being romantic.

Our sex and love life seemed to grind to halt. I was sure that if I "gave in" (which is how I saw it) to more hugging and touching, it would mean the end of our sex life. I pictured two old folks who love to cuddle, but haven't really "done it" for the last 35 years. I wasn't ready to give up my sex life.

There came a time where I was having difficulty getting and maintaining an erection even when Carlin was ready, willing, and able. I was terrified. I thought that I was really going to lose my sex life. Instead I found something quite wonderful. There really *is* more to sex than a hard penis. I found we could play and touch, cuddle and fondle, lick and linger. We still love to have intercourse, but it isn't the be-all and end-all it once was. We don't fight as much because "I want it and she doesn't." Now we both enjoy wanting "it," but the "it" has expanded. Magnetic sex draws us into a whole new dimension of pleasure.

Retirement: A Time to Express Our Manly Magnetic Nature

The andropause and menopause passages involve the descent down the mountain of first adulthood and through the valley below. Its purpose is to prepare us for the ascent up the second mountain so that we can fully engage life's later years, what psychologist Carl Jung called "the afternoon of life."

Much of the discomfort associated with this time of life comes from the growing pains we experience. The degree of pain is proportional to the degree to which we cling to the past and refuse to embrace the future. It can be one of the most challenging times in a relationship and also the most rewarding. This was the case for Ruth and Jeremy.

"It was a bigger disruption to our lives than the birth of our first child," says Ruth, describing her husband Jeremy's retirement. "He had been working since he was a teenager and all of a sudden he has no role, no title, no job definition. He became very dependent on me, almost like a child," she continued, remembering those first few months. "He couldn't think clearly. He lost his initiative, and needed me to show him how things worked around the house. It just wasn't like him. Though we had both worked through most of our married life, the house was always my domain," Ruth acknowledged. "When Jeremy came home, he tried to take over. It's understandable, really. He's used to being in charge, particularly when he is around women."

Ruth described what life had been like for Jeremy. He'd spent 40 years being surrounded by secretaries, research assistants, and waitresses—all female, all focused on being supportive of his needs. He had been the leader, the organizer. Now he didn't have anyone to lead and nothing that needed organizing. All the weight of his changes seemed to fall on his wife.

For Ruth it was a time of stress and turmoil. "I got sick for three months and finally took a trip to visit friends. One told me I ought to leave Jeremy. But I didn't want to do that. I knew he needed to find his own structure and he finally did."

Ruth described how Jeremy came to terms with his emotions. "He joined a men's group and for the first time in his life he began to hear stories of men's pain. One day he came home crying. I'd never seen him cry before. I asked him about it and his response touched my heart. He told me he was thinking about himself when he was nine years old. I could tell he was remembering the pain of what he didn't receive from his father."

For Jeremy it was an opening to a whole new side of himself. Listening to the pain of younger men allowed him to experience his own pain. It also allowed him to share with others his years of experience. He found he had something valuable to offer. "For the first time in my life," said Jeremy, "I really felt I had something of myself that I could give. I could listen to them without judgment. I could hug them with genuine warmth."

Jeremy found that young men would call him on the phone and spend hours talking about their lives and sharing feelings. He would meet with them in coffeehouses and help them sort out their lives over a cup of coffee and a cinnamon roll. He began to visit a man at the local prison through a program that linked inmates with men in the community. "I was afraid I had retired from life when I retired from work," Jeremy confided. "I'm discovering a whole new life opening up for me."

He said that Ruth's support was crucial in helping him get through the initial struggles. He was pretty difficult to live with. He was angry a lot of the time. Often he was demanding and very critical of the things Ruth tried to do to help. "I knew she felt damned if she did and damned if she didn't," Jeremy said. "I wish I could have made it easier on her, but I'm glad we got through it together."

Gender Crossing Is Universal

The process of older men becoming more magnetic in their nature and older women becoming more dynamic seems to be a universal phenomenon. In women we hear about the "postmenopausal zest" that many experience. In men we're just beginning to recognize these changes.

Dr. David Gutmann, professor of psychiatry and education and director of the Older Adult Program at Northwestern University, has been studying human development for over 40 years. He found that in cultures throughout the world there was a gender crossover for men and women.

In evaluating cross-cultural data from around the world, Gutmann says that a significant sex-role turnover takes place as men begin to own, as part of themselves, the qualities of "sensuality, affiliation, and nurturing"—in effect, the "femininity" that was previously repressed and lived out vicariously through their wives. By the same token, Gutmann found the opposite effect in women. They generally become more "unsentimental, assertive, and independent."

As Carlin and I move through this time of life, these are exactly the changes we notice in ourselves and each other. It is the source of our greatest joy and also the source of our greatest conflict.

When I have done something I feel is particularly romantic and caring that Carlin doesn't seem to notice, my feelings get easily hurt. I spend time mulling over a decision about whether we should invite friends over for the holidays. Carlin pushes right ahead and makes the decision for us. I end up feeling left out and angry. Carlin plans a trip to China and is pleased if I want to join her, but seems perfectly happy to make the trip on her own. I feel unneeded.

When I sense conflict between us I often feel it is because she is being too unsentimental, assertive, and independent. I wonder what happened to the nice, sweet, giving woman I married.

Carlin and I often go to the movies. I always want to hold her hand, especially if there is a particularly romantic part. She quickly pulls away. Later she tells me it distracts her from enjoying the movie. We're at a party and I come over to touch her or give her a hug. Later she tells me she feels I'm always checking up on her, not giving her enough space.

She seems to be complaining about my qualities of sensuality, affiliation, and nurturing. She tells me she wonders what happened to her fun-loving, independent husband. I seem so clingy lately.

The real problem, I believe, is that both men and women have difficulty recognizing and accepting these changes. We seem to have two models of relationship for later life. One is to try to hold on to our old roles. The other is to shed our roles completely and take on a unisex model in which each partner tries to divorce him- or herself from sex roles altogether and just be a "human being."

The result is often a relationship that breaks under the stress of rigid sex roles that no longer fit the needs of each person or a relationship in which the partners deny feelings or behaviors associated with traditional sex roles and become "elder twins." Some men try to deny the magnetic qualities that are beginning to emerge and run off with younger women to reassert their traditional masculine sexuality.

When couples complain that the sex has gone out of their relationship, it is often because they don't feel "manly" or "womanly." They develop an asexual relationship, one in which maleness and femaleness are seen as relics from a sexist society and are best done away with. It often serves to relieve the inevitable tensions of a long-term committed relationship, but sacrifices the juicy sensuality that comes from gender differences.

ACTION OPTION

Plan a Reversed Role Date

Plan a sensual evening together during which the woman takes on the dynamic aspects and the man allows himself to enjoy the magnetic dimension. The woman plans the evening. She decides where you will go and what you will do. She also pays for the evening.

At the agreed-upon time, she will pick the guy up, perhaps bring him a small gift. His job is to enjoy the anticipation of waiting for her to arrive. When she does, he can enjoy looking forward to an evening that he does not have to plan.

When you return, she will take charge of creating a sensual mood for the rest of the evening. She might have a bottle of wine chilling and candles burning. She might offer to give him a massage to help him relax.

I think you get the picture. Be creative. When I have done this exercise with couples, many said it was one of the best things they've ever done. He loved being wooed and seduced, and she loved taking the active role. Many couples build this in as a regular part of their lives.

CHAPTER 15

Coming to Peace with the Woman and Reclaiming Our True Roles as Men

We can't be comfortable in intimacy with women because we have never been comfortable in being distant from them.

—Sam Keen

I BELIEVE THE MATERIAL in this chapter is some of the most important and also the most difficult of any in the book. Many of you won't want to hear this at all. I can tell you that it has been the most valuable and useful information I have ever worked with. It has helped me overcome life-long feelings of loneliness and depression. I believe it has allowed me to develop a wonderful relationship with my wife and helped us to remain together after more than 20 years.

I invite you to jump on in, even if the material seems far out. It will require a leap of faith for many, but it may be the best move you have ever made.

Getting in Touch with the Woman Within

Let me tell you a story of how this journey began in my own life. Right around the time I hit 40 I attended a workshop with Carlin. I don't even remember the theme now, but there were about 50 women and 50 men who attended. One of the exercises they did involved the women sitting on the floor in a large circle with the men sitting silently on the outside. The women were free to talk about whatever they wanted: what it meant to be a woman, what they liked and didn't like about men, what they were doing with their lives, and the barriers they felt to being themselves. I sat on the outside with the men, listening closely, fascinated with the depth of their sharing and their ability to talk as though they were alone with each other and there were no men present.

When the women finished it was time for the men to move into the circle and the women to move out. As I moved forward, one of the women in front of me patted the spot on the floor beside her as if to say, "Here, take my seat. I'm leaving." I moved into the circle at the spot she indicated then quickly moved, as though I had sat on a hot burner.

Once again she patted the spot and once again I sat there, then moved again, as she shrugged and went to the outer ring. I immediately broke into tears. All this had occurred in a period of about 20 seconds, just enough time for the women to move out and for the men to move in.

It seemed that nothing had occurred yet, no words had been spoken, and here I was sitting in the circle crying. When I was finally able to talk, I told the other men what had occurred for me in those 20 seconds. A woman had touched a spot on the floor and I had immediately sat there.

For me it was a gesture I had done in some way all my life. It felt like I was forever seeking out a woman so I could "plug into" her energy. Sitting on the spot she had selected was like connecting with the energy source that only a woman possesses, tapping into the very essence of life itself.

Sitting there I felt immediately uncomfortable and compelled to move. I felt that if I didn't move I would die. Her smile, her invitation, and the knowing pat of her hand were also familiar. In the past I would get a glimpse of my own deep need to find my own juice, my own energy. But if a woman insisted, I would feel I had no choice. As Zorba the Greek said to his young friend, "If a woman calls, you must go."

I would follow her lead. I'd done that my whole life, too. Either I would feel drawn magnetically into the force field of a woman and lose myself, or I would resist my desire to merge and melt and would throw up angry barriers and withdraw before I got sucked in.

But finally I sat in my own seat, and something transformative occurred. The best way I can describe the dilemma I had faced all my life is like this: I must tap into the force field of the woman or I will die, but if I sit where she asks, it will kill me. Somewhere inside I felt I must find my own spot, tap into my own energy, even if it meant I would cease to exist. And in that moment I felt a return of an energy I didn't even know was inside me.

—~~—

A number of days after I attended the workshop I had a dream that seemed a continuation of the earlier experience. I was in my bedroom feeling very sad and alone. In the dream I kept being reminded of all the women I had loved who had left me. I thought of my wife and wondered how long I could count on her to stay. I thought of my first wife and when our divorce had become final. I started to cry as I remembered the past. I went all the way back to my first girlfriend and remembered when we broke up. I went back before that and remembered being a child and all the times my mother had been too busy to be there for me, and I cried even more deeply.

When I felt I had cried all my tears I felt lighter, almost peaceful. But I also felt lonely. When will I find the woman who will be there for me? When will I find the one I can count on not to leave me? Just then the floor opened up and I fell through into another room. I looked around and although I didn't recognize where I was, it felt strangely familiar. All of a sudden there appeared a beautiful woman I immediately recognized. She was the Woman in me, the feminine part of my deepest self. "Why did you leave me?" she asked.

I capitalize this Woman to indicate that she is not a flesh-and-blood woman, but someone deeper, larger, and more mysterious. In the depth psychology pioneered by Dr. Carl Jung, this Woman would be called an archetype.

Archetypes operate at a deeper level than what some call our unconscious or less-conscious sides of ourselves. They are dynamic energies in all of us and can influence us in positive or negative ways depending on how well we relate to them. As we will see, the archetype of Woman expresses herself in many ways. In order to have a complete relationship with ourselves and with any woman in our lives, we must develop a relationship with the Woman.

When I took time to tune into these deepest parts of myself, I realized I had spent my whole life looking outside for the Woman that was waiting for me all the time. I had not been abandoned as I had believed all my life, but had actually abandoned *her.* I cried for all the years I had wasted blaming women for not giving me the kind of love I could only get from her. A wise woman once told me that *no one loves anyone the way that everyone wants to be loved.*

When we confuse the love that can come from the women in our lives with the love that can *only* come from the spiritual Woman within, we are in trouble. Part of the journey we begin in midlife and pursue for the rest of our lives is to find and get to know that inner Woman that can guide us to our true selves.

ACTION OPTION

Explore the Woman in You

Write down all the things you know about the Woman in you. Pay special attention to those parts of yourself you have repressed because they weren't manly enough. Write about how you feel about this side of yourself. Share your writing with someone you care about and trust.

Our Woman as Mystical Mom

There is a cartoon I saw recently that shows a young man on one knee in front of a woman, holding her hand and looking up lovingly into her eyes. The caption reads: "Will you marry me . . . and be my Mommy?" Most women who see it laugh deeply with a knowing nod. Most men give an uncomfortable chuckle, like we're seeing something we'd prefer to deny.

There is a deep longing in men to get the kind of loving we had once received as infants from our mothers. All our needs were met without our having to ask. We were fed, kept warm, had our diapers changed, looked at with adoration, cooed to, and nurtured. Who wouldn't want to go back to the Eden of our infancy? Even those of us who didn't get all we had hoped for long for what we know we lacked.

I remember that in my first marriage I was always conflicted about letting my wife nurture me in any way. On the one hand, I wanted it more than anything. On the other hand, I was afraid to receive it. If I let myself have even a little, I was sure I would want more and more. My ultimate fear was that I would cease to be a man, cease even to exist in this world. I would want to crawl up inside her and never come out. Even these thoughts scared me. I rarely let them come to consciousness.

At the time I thought I was having trouble relating to my wife. Who I was really having trouble with was the Woman as Mystical Mom. Why are men so hung up with this Mom archetype? Why are we insatiably hungry for this kind of nurturing at the same time we fear it so much?

There is a biological reality that most males deal with and that most females do not. All of us come out of the body of a woman. Most men will fall in love and have intimate contact with someone of the same sex as the woman out of whose body we emerged. Most women will not. This is a result of the biological reality that most men and women are heterosexual.

Gay men share the reality of coming out of the body of a woman. Since they will become attracted to and fall in love with a male, they share this experience with heterosexual women. Based on my own experience working with gay and straight men, it seems to me that gay men are generally less conflicted about becoming intimate than are straight men. However, all men (and women) must deal with the Woman as Mystical Mom.

When we heterosexual guys get anywhere close to a woman, we recall the sights, smells, touches, sounds, and feel of our mothers. Beyond that we feel the universal draw of Mom—all giving, all nurturing, always there for us in all ways. It's no surprise that we would like that. Who wouldn't? The problem is that like the guy in the cartoon we confuse being married to a woman, with all her fine points as well as flaws, with the mythical Mom of our dreams.

Since I have discovered the Woman I can more readily accept the love and affection that a real woman can give me. I can also accept that I'll never get all that my inner child would like to receive. I've developed a way to get the kind of mothering that I'll never be able to get from a real live woman, even from my mother when she was alive.

I have created an inner Woman that I relate to when I need unconditional love and nurturing, which I still do from time to time. In my inner world she is young, beautiful, and bountiful. At times of trouble I will picture her holding and nurturing me and telling me all the things I need to hear to know things will be all right.

This is one of the things that may sound silly when you read it. I'll tell you, though, that getting in touch with this aspect of the Woman can help us get through some very difficult times. It also helps us get what we need without putting unrealistic pressure on our mates.

The Woman for me is named Rebecca. She has been with me for many years now. She is available 24 hours a day, every day, and will be forever. She always has time for me. There is never any ambivalence when she nurtures me. It is absolutely pure, unconditional love.

ACTION OPTION

Do the Woman-in-You Meditation

Here's what you can do if you would like to get in touch with the Woman in you. If you don't like the term, make up one that you do like, such as the Mystical Mom. Take some time out from whatever you are doing. Find a comfortable place where you won't be disturbed. Sit in a chair that is comfortable, but one that won't put you to sleep.

You may want to record the following or have someone you trust read it to you. Be sure and leave time for you to follow the directions. Speak in a slow, soothing voice.

Close your eyes and take a number of deep breaths. With each breath you breathe in imagine that you are taking in energy from the universe. With each breath you breathe out imagine that this energy is spreading throughout your body. Breathe comfortably and let yourself relax more and more.

Imagine that you are on a bridge with a stream running beneath. You are relaxed and comfortable on the bridge. You might hear the water beneath you, feel your hands on the railing, see leaves in the water as they are gently carried downstream.

I'd like you now to let go of anything that you are carrying that interferes with your being totally present. Imagine that you could throw off the bridge any thoughts, feelings, experiences that draw your attention away from the present moment.

Imagine that you could take each one, gently throw it off the bridge, knowing you can pick it up later if you want to. But now, just let it go.

Breathe easy and relax. Don't worry about doing this right or losing focus. Simply bring your attention back to the bridge and continue on.

Now continue walking across the bridge. When you get to the other side, imagine you find yourself in a place that you love. It can be a place you've actually been to or a place you create now in your mind.

Without thought or effort, let yourself be there now. Take a deep breath and let it out. Good.

Now look around and see what sights you associate with this place.

What sounds do you hear?

If you could touch what you see and hear, how would these things feel?

Are there aromas associated with this place? Breathe deeply and bring them in.

Imagine that you can walk around in this place until you come to a spot that draws your attention. It will feel inviting and comfortable.

When you find it, sit down and relax. You're now going to invite the ever present, all-nurturing, unconditionally loving Woman to join you. She has been waiting for you for a long time. Take a deep breath and let it out. Good.

Look off into the distance. Everything you see, hear, and feel is beautiful. As you look you see something on the horizon. You can't make it out, but you know it's a person.

As the person continues walking you can tell by the walk that she is a woman. Even in the distance she gives off an aura of calm.

As she gets closer you can begin to make out some of her features. You are able to tell some things about her: the color of her hair, how tall she is, how old, the expression on her face.

She looks lovingly at you as she approaches.

She sits down facing you, and you feel enveloped in warmth. You feel safe and loved unconditionally.

She tells you her name and lets you know that she is your Woman and has been waiting for you for a very long time. She knows all the hurts and pains you've experienced in your life. She is aware of all you got or didn't get when you were a child. She will be there for you whenever you want her to be.

You reach out to her and she enfolds you in her arms. You melt into her body and know that you can get what you need here and leave full and replenished.

You say good-bye for now, knowing that you will get to know each other better and better as time goes on.

You walk back to the bridge now, feeling wonderful, relaxed, and free.

Cross over the bridge now. When you do you will find yourself returned to this time and this place. You feel your feet on the floor, your body against the seat. Slowly, gently you open your eyes, feeling relaxed and comfortable.

Don't worry if you weren't able to see, hear, or feel all the things I suggested to you. Some people are better at experiencing different aspects of this meditation. Everyone gets better with practice. I suggest you do this at least once a week. Each time you do, it will become more natural and you will learn more about your Woman. Over time you will be able to go to her when you need all the gifts that she has to offer.

I have used this meditation for many years, and it has helped people work through a variety of issues. Once you learn it, you will find you can adapt it to all kinds of situations. Wouldn't you like to go to a place where everything you see, hear, and feel reflects back to you how worthwhile and wonderful you are? Wouldn't you like to spend time in a place of unconditional love and support?

Well, you can. You only need the willingness to go there and the courage to practice. Believe me, the payoff will be more than you ever expected. All I can say is try it. You'll be glad you did.

—~—

Our Dream Lover Woman

Have you ever looked at a woman that you love and care about and found yourself comparing her to someone else? I know I have. Many of us heterosexual men are never able to develop a healthy, intimate relationship with a woman because we can never find "the one" who can satisfy all our requirements. Others of us seem to sabotage good relationships because we start looking elsewhere for someone more exciting and attractive. Does this sound familiar to you?

What I believe we are really looking for is our Dream Lover Woman. She is the woman of our dreams and she *is* sensational. Many of us spend our lives searching the earth for her. We die feeling we've never found the woman we really want. I know where she is. Are you interested in finding her?

It helps if we know something about her makeup. She is one part mother, one part first girlfriend, one part sex symbol of our youth, and one part what's missing in us. When we get anywhere close to a woman in the flesh-and-blood world that resonates with these qualities, we are drawn as a moth to a flame.

Let me tell you about my Dream Lover.

From my mother I got the memory of large, soft breasts that nurtured me as an infant. As I grew up she told me repeatedly that I could do anything I wanted and become successful at anything I tried. She was successful in the business world and was respected by most men.

My first girlfriend was named Linda. She was short with straight, jet black hair. Her appearance was cute and pixielike. Though she was short, she was well endowed. She kissed like she could never get enough and was always drawing the attention of other guys.

The sex symbol of my youth was Brigitte Bardot, the French bombshell who starred in a movie called *And God Created Woman.* Talk about getting hooked on an archetypal sex symbol. Wow! I was 13 or 14 at the time when her movie was showing at the local theater. You had to be over 18 to go in, but my buddies and I knew we had to get a look. We sneaked in, and I don't know about them, but my life was never the same.

From Bardot I got a taste for exotic, sexual women. I also got a heavy dose of illicit sex. My psyche was shaped by the belief that sex is most exciting if there are elements of risk and danger. Her face and her body are indelibly stamped on my brain nearly 45 years after my hour-and-a-half encounter on the big screen.

What I always felt was missing in me was being able to make other people's eyes turn when I walked into the room. Since I've always been short, I never felt like I stood out. My Dream Lover is a head turner. When she walks into a room, heads swivel. When she talks, people listen.

Exploring this archetype of the Dream Lover Woman has given me great insight into understanding the kinds of women I am drawn to, usually outside my full consciousness. To put it all together, my Dream Lover Woman is short, dark, exotic, and sexy, with large, inviting breasts. She has absolute faith in who I am and my ability to be successful in the world. Her kisses are passionate and fiery, and there is always a quality of danger surrounding her.

Though she is totally committed to me, all men and many women are drawn to her. There is something dangerous and illicit about her that both frightens me and turns me on.

Quite a package, am I right? Do you get a feel (no pun intended) for the kind of woman who attracts me? Can you understand why no woman can ever live up to my Dream Lover Woman?

I have found we need to acknowledge our Dream Lover Woman. She is very real, but she is not flesh and blood. She lives in a different world. Keeping her secret not only deprives us of the pleasure of her company, it keeps us from fully enjoying the company of other women. We can visit her there in her world and enjoy all the wonderful aspects of her being. But if we continue to look for her in this world we will damage every relationship we will ever have with a woman.

ACTION OPTION

Explore the Four Aspects of Your Dream Lover

Write down the four elements that go into your Dream Lover Woman. Detail the aspects that come from your mother, your first girlfriend, the sex symbol of your youth, and the undeveloped parts of yourself. Notice what feelings arise as you do this exercise. Share your experience with someone close to you.

The 10,000-Year-Old War Cry of Men Attacking Woman

As I suggested earlier and want to make crystal clear here, when we moved from being hunter-gatherers to becoming herders and farmers we began a journey toward what we know as civilization. It has been a journey that has clearly been devastating to the wilderness and to the natural resources of the planet. It has also been damaging to women. It has been particularly destructive to men.

Let's look at the key roles that allow us to feel useful, worthwhile, valuable—in short, the things that give us the internal experience of being men.

1. The hunting way of life—gone.
2. The importance of each man for group protection—gone.
3. Our support in men's groups and ability to initiate, guide, and teach young men—gone.
4. Extended time to play with, nurture, and listen to our children—gone.
5. The spiritual nourishment we have always received from the wild—gone.

The more that these roles have shrunk over the last 10,000 years, the smaller the archetypal Man has become in relationship to the Woman. The smaller we've become, the angrier we've gotten. Though the soul of the Man may have gotten smaller, the bodies of men are still larger than women's. Though we may have lost our hunting role, we have retained the hunter's ability to unleash all his power, cunning, and strength to kill another.

I believe that men have been at war with the Woman for the last 10,000 years and don't even know it. We feel threatened by this huge Woman and try to protect ourselves by cutting her down to size. Women feel terrorized and brutalized. The first step in ending our war with the Woman is to admit that out of our weakness we have become tyrants.

We need to take responsibility for what the Man has done, and continues to do, to the Woman.

ACTION OPTION

Listen to a Woman's Pain

Seek out a woman you trust and who trusts you. Ask her to share the experiences in her life in which angry men have harmed her physically or emotionally. Pay close attention to the feelings that come up in you as you listen. Ask her to tell you about other women she's known who have been similarly harmed. Ask her forgiveness on behalf of yourself as a man and on behalf of the other wounded men in the world who continue to harm women.

Coming to Peace with the Woman

If we are going to end the war with the Woman that has taken such a huge toll on the lives of women, men, and children, there are a number of simple steps we must take.

1. We need to recognize and accept the fact that there has been a war going on.

In order to change anything, we first have to accept that it exists. As long as we deny the process, we remain stuck.

2. We need to take responsibility for our part in the war on the Woman.

One of the most pervasive and confusing things I have seen in all men, to a greater or lesser degree, is our pervasive anger. I have spent years in therapy trying to get at the root of the problem in my relationships with my wives, girlfriends, and mother. As deep as I went and as much healing as I know occurred, there was always more that seemed to be just out of my awareness.

Now I know I have been at war with the Woman. It's a war I never chose, but one I have participated in fighting. I am ready to end my involvement in it. I'm ready to stop being "mad as hell" and blaming women for my pain. I'm also ready to stop seeing women in my life as responsible for making me feel better.

3. We need to recognize that our anger at the Woman comes from our fear that she will destroy us because she is so much bigger than the Man.

As individuals we all have to recognize that a lot of the fear we carry toward women results from our first seeing them as very large mothers who had complete control over our lives. Collectively we need to recognize that for the last 10,000 years the Man has been looking up at the very large Woman, who also seemed to have control of us.

4. Accept that the Man will never be able to become equal again with the Woman by trying to cut her down to size.

For the last 10,000 years we have been running around like deranged mental midgets, grabbing at the Woman and trying to bring her down to our level. No matter what the Man has done, though, the Woman won't be permanently diminished. No matter how many women we harmed, we never feel like men. No matter how many other men we killed, it will never make us whole.

5. The only way the Man can regain his stature is by returning to his roots.

Sir Winston Churchill once said of Americans that we always do the right thing—after we've tried everything else. The same thing holds true for the Man. We've done everything we could to regain our equality with the Woman except the only thing that will work.

It's time we grew up. It's time that we reclaimed our ancient roles and adapted them to our modern times. Remember that I said the steps would be simple; I didn't say they would be easy.

6. We need to learn how to hunt again.

In this context I'm talking about "the hunt" as an archetype for a way of making our living. In order to live, something else must die. If we are meat eaters, animals must die. Even if we are vegetarians we interfere with the natural life cycles of plants. We can't escape the killing.

However, we need to find a way of living that, like ancient hunting, is in balance with our own deepest desires and with the natural world. We need work that nourishes the spirit, not just the body. We need work that is truly valuable to ourselves, our families, our communities, and our planet. We need work that takes only what is necessary from the world. We need work that does not pollute, but returns all our waste products to be recycled by nature.

In order to feel connected again to the natural world, I recommend we go out into nature. Look at nature through the eyes of our ancestral hunter-gatherers. If we had to rely on the natural world for our nourishment (and in the larger sense we all do), what is there to eat? What plants are edible? How would we kill an animal if we needed its meat to survive? How would we shelter ourselves in the wild? Where would we find water?

These are some of the questions Carlin and I had when we attended our first wilderness classes with Tom Brown, an expert on wilderness survival who teaches about all aspects of living in balance with nature. We got answers to these questions and many more. We left the classes with a much better sense of what it means to be so much a part of nature that we don't feel like outsiders.

ACTION OPTION

Change the Way You Make a Living

Talk to a buddy about the way you make your living. Discuss the ways your work does or does not contribute to the well-being of the planet. Take one action that would make your contribution more positive and one action that would reduce the negative impact you have on the planet.

7. We need to take responsibility for group protection.

Nowadays all too many men carry guns to protect ourselves. Our children, mostly young males, bring them to school to act like men and for personal protection. We install burglar alarms in our cars and in our houses to keep others from stealing our property.

But that's not the same as protecting the collective. Even our armies have become instruments for spreading and supporting our corporate interests rather than truly protecting the citizens. That needs to change.

Group protection needs to be a role that we each take upon ourselves. For some of us, that may be going to a trouble spot in the world to help warring groups of men sit down and talk to each other.

For others it may involve joining a community watch program to patrol our streets and make our towns and cities safer for all men, women, and children.

ACTION OPTION

Create a Safer School Environment

Take a trip to your local high school. Talk to the administration, teachers, and students about what can be done to create a safe environment for children. Join with other men to help provide group support.

8. We need to initiate our boys into manhood.

Throughout human history one of the main responsibilities of men has been to initiate boys. This need is even more important in modern times. As discussed in chapter 6, in the first cross-cultural study of manhood, anthropologist David Gilmore found that becoming a man is a process that must be achieved through some sort of stressful series of tests. Some of these tests of manhood are bloody and violent. Others are more gentle. But all require a test of some kind, and in all cases older men teach and guide the youths. There is a recognition that boys cannot become men without a ritual initiation and that older men must be involved.

The escalation of violence we continue to see displayed by young males results, to a great degree, from a lack of initiation rites. It's as though there is a fire that begins to burn inside a young man when he reaches the age of eight or nine. Somewhere inside he knows that it is time to begin preparations for his transition to manhood. He is primed to wait for the male elders who traditionally came and took the boy out of his mother's keeping and begin his training.

But the men never come, and the boy's disappointment and anger begin to build. The violence we see in our schools and in our streets is an expression of the rage that many young men feel at being abandoned by their elders. It is also an attempt to create their own initiation, one that is dangerous and requires a test of bravery. However, without the guidance of the male elders, all that is left is the violent attempt to prove that they are men.

ACTION OPTION

Plan a Modern-Day Initiation

Get together with a group of male friends and talk about the need to initiate boys into men. Discuss the things that you would have needed from older men as you grew up. Discuss what experiences young men need today to feel that they are becoming adults. Detail the elements of a modern-day initiation.

9. We need to spend more time with our children throughout their lives.

Fatherhood is one of the hallmarks of human evolution. In every other animal species, males contribute very little to the lives of mothers and their babies. Sometimes all they contribute is sperm. Mothers and offspring are the social unit, and the males hang out together on the periphery.

But as we evolved the human brain got bigger and bigger until it was difficult for us big-headed creatures to pass through our mothers' birth canals. The solution was that human babies were born with immature brains and thus required many years of support and learning before we were ready to survive in the world on our own. We needed support from both our mothers and our fathers.

In recent times we seem to be returning to an earlier evolutionary pattern in which fathers were less involved with their children than were mothers. As a society we seem much more concerned that absent fathers pay child support than we are to ensure that mothers support a dad's visitation rights. Fathers are often left feeling that they are only needed for their money. Many women now feel quite comfortable raising children on their own without the involvement of a man.

However, the ancient need of children for the things that a mother and a father can offer have not changed. Our children need both of us more than ever. They need more from us than a kiss at bedtime or a ride to their baseball games on the weekend. There is no such thing as quality time if it is so short that our hearts can't settle, relax, and have time to open up.

10. We need to spend more time in the wilderness.

If you ask people in the developed world, most of us would say that we enjoy spending time in nature. We often remember times and places from our childhood where we played outside and were overcome with the joy and peace of being away from our domesticated lives at home.

I believe that this is not only a universal desire, but a universal need. Spending time in the wilderness, away from things human, is as necessary for our health and well-being as eating the right foods and getting the right exercise.

ACTION OPTION

Meditate in the Wilderness

Go someplace where there is very little sign of humans. Try to be in this place for at least three days. It will be worth it. Set up your camp and look around. Notice how different you feel to be surrounded by what is wild and natural. During your time in camp, take time to meditate on what the wilderness has to teach you about your life and the life of the planet. Ask for guidance from the spirit of the wilderness on what you can bring back to your day-to-day life that would help the human community on the earth.

I hope you have gotten a new understanding of the steps we need to take to end our battle with the Woman and to learn to appreciate ourselves as men. When we reenergize these roles in our lives, we will feel like healthy, powerful, whole men again. As we live more in the fullness of our masculinity, we will be less threatened by the feminine principle in the world and more at home with the Woman. As we embrace the archetypal feminine, we will be able to have more healthy relationships with the women in our lives.

CHAPTER 16

Developing and Maintaining Intimacy

Love and intimacy are at the root of what makes us sick and what makes us well, what causes sadness and what brings happiness, what makes us suffer and what leads to healing.

—Dean Ornish, M.D.

The Healing Power of Love and Intimacy

We all know that having close friends and an intimate partner makes all our pains and illnesses easier to bear. There is also new and exciting research that shows that love and intimacy can actually heal the body as well as the spirit.

Men die of heart disease more often than from any other cause. We are learning about the importance of such things as diet, exercise, and stress on whether we live long and well or die too soon. But our hearts are not just physical pumps that send blood throughout our bodies. We have an emotional heart, a passionate heart, and a spiritual heart.

Nourishing the nonphysical aspects of our being is just as important as seeing that the physical is being nourished. We know now that there really is not a separation between the physical, emotional, and spiritual aspects of our being. They are related to each other. Our intimate relationships are the places where all aspects of our lives can come together.

When we have love and intimacy in our lives, we are healthy. When they are lacking, we are sick.

We all know people who have lost a loved one and then quite literally die of a broken heart. Studies show that when a man's partner dies after a long-term relationship, he is likely to die within the next five years. There are also many cases where a loving relationship prolongs the healthy life span of men.

- In 1994 British researchers who tracked 8,000 men for 11 years found that unmarried guys had a greater risk of dying young. Men who became divorced during the course of the study were four times more likely to die than men who stayed married.
- A 1998 Danish study found that men with colon cancer survive longer if they're married.
- In 1999 Canadian researchers found that elderly people who are married are far less likely to suffer from dementia or to be institutionalized than unmarried people.

Some argue that married men engage in more healthy practices and refrain from more unhealthy practices than single men. That is undoubtedly true. The key factor, however, seems to be the healthy benefits of love and intimacy. This was the surprising conclusion of more than 20 years of research by Dr. Dean Ornish, who was the first physician to prove that heart disease could actually be reversed by changing our lifestyles.

Though most people paid attention to Dr. Ornish's focus on a low-fat diet and exercise as important factors in helping people live long and well, they neglected his findings on love and intimacy. "I am not aware of any other factor in medicine—not diet, not smoking, not exercise, not stress, not genetics, not drugs, not surgery," says Ornish, "that has a greater impact on our quality of life, incidence of illness, and premature death from all causes."

Love and Intimacy in a Long-Term Committed Relationship

I believe very strongly that before we can really have a deep relationship with an intimate partner, we have to come to peace with the archetypal Woman. However, it's also true that we can't learn much about the archetypal Woman until we stay in a relationship with a partner long enough to know them well enough to become deeply intimate.

The more we learn about the Woman, the more we will learn about the women in our lives, and vice versa. Although there are some things we can say, generally, about healing our intimate relationships, the process is always very personal. It is a loving, moving, sometimes painful, and always mysterious dance between two people.

Although I will share my own experiences as a heterosexual male, I believe that a good deal of what I say will be helpful to all kinds of intimate relationships. When I talk to my gay friends and clients about their intimate relationships, most of the issues are identical to those that heterosexual couples experience. There are discussions about communication problems, jealousy, fear of aging, decreasing stamina, and loss of sex drive. There are also the joys of intimacy, building a life together, and growing old with someone you love.

There are also significant differences. In addition to the grief all of us experience as we deal with the losses of those we love through the years, gay men also must deal with the devastation and deaths of their peers as a result of AIDS. Many have already gone through the death of an intimate partner or are living with a partner who is HIV-positive.

Since our society does not recognize the union of most gay couples, many have to go through the additional trauma of denied access to their partner because they are not "family." I know a man who had been in an intimate partnership for over 20 years. When his partner got sick and was in the last days of his life, he was not allowed to visit him in the hospital because the dying man's family didn't want him to be present.

These kinds of stresses can draw some couples closer together. They can also tear others apart. Whatever effect they have on couples, gay men have an added level of stress that comes from our society's outmoded practices.

ACTION OPTION

Meditate on Love and Loss

Take some time for yourself. Find a comfortable place where you will not be disturbed. Close your eyes and take in a number of deep breaths. Let your mind and body relax. In your mind's eye imagine yourself in the center of a circle surrounded by all those you love.

Imagine that each person is bathed in light, as though a spotlight was shining down on your loved one. Feel the warmth and comfort of having those you love all around you. Now count to 10 and imagine that one of the lights goes out and that person disappears. Notice how you feel.

Once again count to 10 and watch as another light goes out and another loved one leaves. Continue this process until there is only one light remaining. It is the person you love the most. Watch as their light begins to dim. You try and reach the person, but are told you are not part of the family and cannot come in. Be aware of how you feel.

Count to 10 in your mind and watch as the final light goes out and you are alone. Be aware of how you feel. If there is anything you would have liked to have said to a loved one or anything you would liked to have done, commit yourself to making it happen now. At some point in time, all the lights go out. We never know when it will happen to us or those we love.

—∞—

As I write this, Carlin and I have been married for 21 years. As I've said, we had each been married twice before and have maintained to each other, as well as to our friends and family, that this was our last marriage. It really was going to be "until death do us part." There have been many times we weren't sure we could keep that agreement.

I've come to see that developing, maintaining, and growing with an intimate relationship is the graduate school of life. It may be the most difficult graduate program on the face of the planet, as divorce statistics show. Even those of us who stay together over long periods of time are not necessarily still intimate and growing. I believe the rewards are worth it *if*—and it's a big *if*—we learn how to have a successful relationship.

I believe that learning to have a successful intimate relationship is not something that is programmed into our genes. It requires healthy and loving parents, siblings and other relatives who are secure in their own lives, a healthy community that understands and supports intimacy, and the skills to put intimacy into practice. It's no wonder that most of our relationships are in trouble. I don't know about you, but most of those things were missing in my life.

—∞—

ACTION OPTION

Reflect on Your Intimate Relationships

Write down the names of the people with whom you have had long-term intimate partnerships. With each person, write about the positive aspects of the relationship and the negative aspects. Next, write about the positive things you received from each of your parents and the negative things you received.

Finally, make a list of the positive things you learned about intimacy from your parents. Make a commitment to bring more of these things into your present relationship. Make a list of the negative things you learned about intimacy from your parents and make a commitment to leave those things behind. Remember that most of what we learn is through our parents' actions, not from what they say about intimacy.

—∞—

After the Children Leave

Like many couples, Carlin and I have spent a good deal of our adult lives raising children. We each first married in our early 20s, raised children, divorced, and raised children on our own. We each had short second marriages before we met and married each other. We prided ourselves on having grown emotionally so that we could truly appreciate a healthy relationship. We had worked out a lot of our childhood issues that had caused problems in our early marriages and looked forward to a joyful, lifelong partnership.

We enjoyed and worked hard at our respective careers, shared housework (though she still did the majority of it), raised our last two children together, and then slowly, imperceptibly at first, began to lose our way. We knew about the stress of the empty-nest syndrome. What do you do when so much energy is devoted to child raising and all of a sudden the children are gone? But that didn't really seem to apply to us. We had both been involved in child rearing for most of our adult lives, but had also had careers that nourished us and to which we were devoted.

It wasn't so much that we were reacting to the nest being empty of children, but more that it now was full of us. We both seemed to be going through a major change time. We were reexamining our careers, where we wanted to live, and who we were as individuals and as a couple. We realized that with the children gone, we had never had so much of our intimate energy directed at each other.

It was new territory for both of us. In the families we grew up in, our parents were divorced long before the last child was grown. We both had aunts and uncles whose marriages lasted more than 50 years and only ended when one of the partners died. But they seemed to have lost their passion and playfulness along the way. They seemed to be together more out of habit than from desire.

We were convinced that we were too smart to let our marriage drift apart or grow stale. After all, we had learned our lessons from our previous marriages. Besides that, we were both therapists and knew all the danger signs of a marriage in trouble and how to keep from falling out of love.

What we didn't know was that second-half relationships were very different from those in the first half and that no matter how well trained you are or how good you are at helping others, it doesn't give you immunity from having your own problems. In fact, as we learned to our dismay, being a therapist can make seeing potential problems *more* difficult. It was easy to believe that we knew too much to have problems, that we could get ourselves out of any difficulties, and that we didn't need help from outside because we were the experts.

The early warning signs were easy to dismiss. We laughed less and took less time to play and have fun. We attributed that to the demands and excitement of our jobs. There were more disagreements over little things that left us feeling misunderstood and alone. But these were little things after all, not to be taken too seriously or worried about too much. Our sex life was less passionate, more routine, and less frequent. But we were getting older. We couldn't expect to be as frisky as we were when we were in our 20s or when we first got together.

Later I began to feel unappreciated and criticized. It seemed that I was always in hot water for some small infraction. I'd leave my clothes out or forget to clean off the counter. I'd break a lightbulb and take too long to get it fixed. I felt like I was getting criticized for the least little thing. "What the hell is going on?" I'd ask myself. "I've never hit her. I don't drink too much. I'm not on drugs. I don't run around with other women. I bring home decent money. What's she complaining about? So I forget a thing or two or get upset occasionally. I'm human. I'm not a machine. I know lots of women who would give anything to have a guy like me. Carlin used to think I was great. Now she acts like I'm out to get her."

Where I felt unappreciated and criticized, Carlin felt attacked and blamed. She was also devastated by my mood swings and my up-and-down behavior. "One of the main things that attracted me to you in the beginning was your 'up' energy and what I saw as your joy for life," Carlin told me, "but over the last few years things have changed."

When Carlin was finally able to convince me to go into therapy, she wrote a letter to my counselor telling her what had changed over the years.

> Now he's more often angry, accusing, argumentative and blaming. What drives me crazy is that he can be nice one minute then explode into a rage the next. One minute he fixes me with a look so intense and cold that it scares me, the next minute he is buying me flowers, sending me cards and loving notes, and is smiling and enthusiastic. I never know which man I'm going to encounter.
>
> I feel like a clam that begins to trust and open up and then is hit with a stick and snaps shut. I have told him over and over that I can only close and open so many times before I'm not willing to risk getting hurt again. I am fairly content to find my joy and play with friends, my work and in other creative activities. I haven't the slightest interest in an affair, but I do have a great desire to have a supportive, easy and loving relationship with Jed and to enjoy life with him.
>
> I am desperately tired of being blamed for his pain. I think I can still revive my feelings for him, but I need to see actions, not just hear words. I long to be cherished and loved. I feel like I've done what I can do and it's now up to him.

It was clear to me that we were both unhappy and in pain, but I didn't know how to break out of it. It seemed to me that if she was more appreciative and accepting, then things could begin to improve. I would alternately long for the woman I remembered early in our relationship and fantasize about finding a woman who wasn't trying to change me, but liked me the way I was. I sensed that Carlin felt I needed to be kinder and more consistently loving before things would improve.

At times I felt we were like hurt children, facing each other red-faced, with our hands on our hips, shouting in our loneliness and pain: "You love me first, then I'll love you back." "No! You have to love *me* first, then I'll love you back." "Me first." "No, me first." "No, me first." "No . . . " It felt like a downward spiral, an iron web we could not break. We were going down together and couldn't seem to save ourselves.

ACTION OPTION

Create a Vision of Intimacy with Your Partner

Find a time when you and your partner can have some quiet moments together. Talk to your partner about the joys of your lives when you first met. Share your memories of the good times you have experienced over the years. Be open to your partner telling you about his or her experiences.

Now talk about how things have been in recent years. Pay particular attention to the joyful experiences that have continued, but also the negative behaviors that may have crept into the relationship. Share with your partner your vision of how you would like your relationship to be and learn about your partner's vision. Commit yourselves to putting that vision into practice. Seek out a health care professional you can both trust if you have trouble doing it yourselves.

Seeing a Therapist: Why Is It So Difficult for Us Guys?

After struggling for many years with my emotional ups and downs, as I mentioned earlier, I finally decided it was time to follow Carlin's advice and seek professional help. You might think that a therapist would recognize the importance of getting help and get it when he needed it.

I'm a man first and a therapist second. Like most men I have difficulty asking for help, and even more difficulty asking for help from someone I don't know who is in an authority position. From the time we fought on the playgrounds of our grammar schools, we learned to keep our feelings to ourselves and not let ourselves show weakness and fear to others.

I think the main reason I went (who am I kidding, the only reason I went) was to please my wife. I sensed that she was getting to the end of her rope and that I'd better show her I was trying, or I might lose her.

I truly did not want to lose my marriage or my connections to our family. For most of our relationship I had taken Carlin's presence pretty much for granted. After the initial courtship when I wasn't really sure she wanted to be with me, I generally felt secure. We loved each other, and I naively thought that love would always be enough to keep our relationship going.

However, once I was able to reach out for help I could see there was much room for improvement and that it needed to start with me. The therapist said there were many treatment options that included medications, herbs, exercise, dietary changes, and cognitive behavior therapy. She said she favored a multiple approach that we would tailor to fit my specific needs. She also emphasized that we were partners in the process. She didn't believe in being the "expert" that told the "sick person" what to do. She didn't even consider me sick. She said some of my difficulties were from the type of genetic makeup I was born with, some from early childhood experiences, some from my past relationships, some from my present relationship with Carlin, and a lot from the way I was thinking about myself and the way I tended to deal with stress in my life.

For the first time I felt I had a professional ally I could work with. I didn't feel so alone, and although I still felt some shame that as a mental health professional I was having problems, I knew I was ready to move ahead.

ACTION OPTION

Discuss Your Fears About Counseling

Talk to your partner about your relationship. Talk about times in the past, if any, when you had been in couples counseling. Pay particular attention to the positive and negative memories you have of those experiences. Discuss the positive things you might get if you were in counseling together now. Discuss your fears of being in counseling. Get clear with your partner about the circumstances that might be present in your relationship that would induce you to go to counseling.

Relationships are the most complex and interesting things in the world. They never stay the same. They are always changing, either for better or for worse. We long to feel nourished by their goodness and are devastated if they do not deliver all that we hope for.

All Intimate Relationships Are Different and All Intimate Relationships Are the Same

In the 37 years I have worked with couples to improve their relationships I have found that each couple is unique. There is no set formula I can offer that says, "Here, if you do *this,* your relationship will improve." However, I have found that all relationships have things in common. We all want to feel safe and know that disagreements won't end in violence. We all want to feel secure and know that we can trust our partner. We all want to feel valued for who we are. We all want to love and be loved. We all want freedom to grow as individuals. We all want our relationship to grow as our needs change through the years.

Men handle this in different ways. Some of us get ulcers, have heart attacks, or develop other serious illnesses. Others go back and forth between their wives and other women. Some live a normal family life on the surface and a sexual life that is kept hidden. One man is a loving husband and father on family time, but on his own time he goes to sex clubs and seeks out prostitutes.

We may get up late at night and turn our computers on as we seek sexual sites where we can fulfill any fantasy that turns us on. In cyberspace our "partner" is available 24 hours a day, will engage in any kind of sexual behavior we can imagine, and never says no, and we never have to worry about being arrested or getting a sexually transmitted disease. It's no wonder that sex makes up the major component of online business.

Some men and their partners seek out counseling. I've seen over 10,000 of these couples in the years I've been working. By the time a couple comes to see me they are often shell-shocked and demoralized. They often feel their only choices are to get out or accept a marriage that is vacant and lifeless.

For many of us these destructive patterns have gone on for so long they seem like second nature. No matter how bad things are, humans are so adaptable that we can get used to just about anything. We gradually give up hope of finding something better and become habituated to things as they are.

We quite literally become addicted to our pain. It becomes familiar. We wrap it around us like a security blanket. Like hostages, we become dependent on our captors. We come to see our partner as both our jailer and the only one we can turn to for survival. Breaking free, seeking health, comes to be seen as dangerous. The very thing that could turn things around for us is seen as alien and destructive, and the patterns that are killing us are seen as our only hope.

Down-to-Earth Help for Improving Your Relationship

Whether your relationship is on the brink of destruction or just needs a little fine-tuning to keep it running well for the rest of your life, these steps will help you. They are based on the thousands of clients I have seen over the years as well as what I've learned with my wife, Carlin. Some of the steps may speak to you more strongly than others. Take what you need and leave the rest.

1. All relationships need nourishment. Nourish your own.

Like plants, relationships need to be protected and nourished. Like a good gardener, we need to keep "weeds" out of our relationships. There are many pressures that can do harm to our relationships, and we need to be aware of them and remove them before they cause problems.

One of our friends owns a restaurant, and we would often gather there in the evenings. Over time it became apparent that our friend was paying special attention to one of the young waitresses. Another buddy noticed, took our friend aside, and alerted him to the danger. He began treating her like an employee again and headed off a problem before it occurred.

During our lives there are three key relationships that need to be nourished. The first is our relationship to ourselves, the second is our relationship to our partners, the third is our relationship to our families and communities. At different times of our lives more attention may go to one or the other, but all need nourishment.

My wife and I found that it was difficult during the years we were raising children to take time for ourselves or nourish our relationship. Once the children left home, we found we had gotten out of practice. It was like we were adolescents again, fumbling around. I wanted her to love me, and I wanted to let her know I loved her, but I felt awkward.

In the second half of life you may need to treat your relationship as if it were new. You may need to court your partner, find new ways to get to know her, and let her see sides of you that may have been hidden over the years. If it has been the woman who has taken the lead in nourishing the relationship in the first half, you may need to be the one to take the lead in the second half. If she was someone new you wanted to have a relationship with, what would you do? Get creative. Have fun.

2. Be sure you are nourishing yourself.

One of the best things a man can do for his relationship with his partner is to make sure his relationship with himself is healthy and growing. When's the last time you did something nice for yourself? In the hustle and bustle of our busy lives we sometimes put ourselves at the bottom of the priority list.

A relationship can only be as healthy as the people who make it up. Be sure you are taking care of yourself as much as you would take care of the person in the world that you care about the most.

3. Be sure you are nourishing your relationships with friends and community.

My wife tells me that one of the best things I ever did for our relationship was join my men's group. We often put a lot of pressure on our partners to fulfill all our emotional needs, particularly as we get older. Having a group of guys I can share my feelings with has allowed me to be less needy at home.

It's important that we have more than one intimate relationship in our lives. Most women have a number of close friends that they confide in and receive support from. Most of us guys have no one. The result is that when we're having difficulties in our relationship, we feel totally alone. I believe that one of the primary reason a man turns to another woman in his later years is that he's looking for more emotional support in his life.

We need to be sure that we have other supports than just our partners. For me, men's groups have been a source of a great deal of care and nurturing. When I feel there are many sources for love in my life, I feel I have more to give to my relationship.

4. All relationships go through pain as they grow. Listen to the pain and act on what you hear.

No relationship can grow without pain. Those of us who want a relationship that is always pain free will always be disappointed in love. If we think that pain and problems are a sign that there is something wrong with our relationship and that we need to find another one that feels better, we will send ourselves on an endless search.

Problems and pain are part of every relationship. It seems to be one of those laws of life. Just as physical pain is the body's way of letting us know that we need to pay attention, relationship pain alerts us to tune into our partnership.

Pain tells us that something has occurred that needs attention *now.* You may feel it when your wife invites her family for a visit without telling you. You may feel it when she doesn't take time to listen when you're telling her about stress at work.

Most of us are trained to ignore or minimize physical pain, and most of us are trained to ignore relationship pain. Don't do it! The first step in healing our pain is to notice that we feel hurt. If we are not aware that something is wrong, we can't do anything to fix it. Once we are aware that we feel hurt, we need to talk our partners.

There are two common ways we tell our partners about our pain that *do not* work very well. I call them "You" statements and "Why" questions.

"You" statements focus the problem on our partners. They are a way of hiding from our pain. They sound like this: "You are always inviting people over without asking me. You never consider my feelings. You never listen to me. You just don't care."

Sound familiar? Notice that all the statements point at the other person. When we're on the other end of the "You" statements we usually feel scolded and blamed.

In relationship communications, I have found that questions are usually ways of hiding feelings rather than requests for information. They often go together with "You" statements: "Why are you always doing this to me?" "Don't you know I have work to do tonight?" "Why don't you ever take an interest in my work?" "How can you be so inconsiderate?"

Have you ever heard yourself asking questions like these? Can you sense the difference between the question I just asked you and the ones in the previous paragraph? Here I really *am* looking for information. I really want to know if you have heard yourself speaking in the way I describe. The other kinds of question are really covers for "You" statements.

So what does work? We need to tell our partners about our pain. We need to let them know that what they do affects us without blaming them for the hurts that we feel. "I" statements focus on us. They tell our partner what is going on inside us. "I" statements are good. The more we use them, the better communication we will have. But they are often difficult to use when we are under stress.

Sometimes I can actually use a good "I" statement when I feel hurt: "I feel disappointed that you invited your aunt to visit without talking to me. I feel left out. I was looking forward to having time just for the two of us."

More often when we feel hurt, the most we can say is "ouch." Under pressure, most of us are not eloquent speakers. Just making a sound that something is wrong may be the best we can do. Whatever we can do, we need to notice our pain and let our partners know what's going on inside of us.

The more we are able to do this, the more alive our relationships will be. The less we do it, the more energy will be lost from our relationships. Eventually, like a tire with a puncture, our relationships will go flat.

Most of us don't want that. Like anything else that is important in life, we need to practice if we want relationships that work.

5. Learn the difference between being receptive and being reactive.

One of the great difficulties we have in discussing our hurts and disappointments with our partners is that we find it very difficult to be receptive rather than reactive. I can't tell you how many times Carlin has tried to tell me something that she is concerned about when before she can finish, I am already reacting defensively.

Being receptive is not an easy practice for most of us to master. We are much better at going on the offensive than listening to what our partners are trying to say to us. Being receptive means listening closely, with openness and love. It does *not* mean closing down while we smile, nod our heads, and say, "Yes dear, yes dear."

I have found that the more receptive we are, the more secure we become. I have also found that the more secure we are, the more receptive we are able to be. In our earlier years we often equated being receptive with being "wimpy" and unmanly. In fact, being receptive is a mark of manly strength. The more we cultivate it, the better we feel about ourselves and the healthier our relationships become.

6. Learn that listening with attention and care is not the same as agreeing with what is being said.

Somehow many of us have gotten the idea that if we listen without responding, it means that we are agreeing with everything the other person is saying. I've found that one of the greatest gifts that one person can give another is to listen to him or her. When we are heard there is a kind of warmth that runs through our bodies. We feel embraced and cared for.

I often have to remind myself, when I am listening to Carlin say something that stirs strong emotions in me, to take a deep breath and just listen. I don't need to defend myself. This is just her point of view, not something I have to challenge. If I can listen with an open heart I know it will help our communication and improve our relationship.

Once our partners feel heard, they are much more receptive to hearing our points of view. A great deal of the pain and conflict that occurs in relationships is because we haven't been able to hear each other. A good deal of what I do as a therapist is just to listen to a person with an open mind and an open heart. This is a skill we can all acquire and which will improve with practice.

7. Learn to listen to your partner's emotions without being overwhelmed.

We've all seen it, in our friends, on TV, or in our own relationships. Our partners are upset about something and become emotional. We withdraw behind a newspaper, the TV, or the computer.

The less responsive we become, the more upset and emotional they become, and the more we withdraw. Sound familiar? Women often complain, "I can never get through to him." Men often complain, "I can't take your constant criticism."

In order to break the pattern, we need to understand what's really going on. Recent research has shown that those who withdraw in the face of strong emotion are actually feeling *flooded* with feelings. Contrary to the belief that women are more emotional than men, men are more emotionally sensitive—we react to emotional situations more strongly—but we often keep our emotions inside.

One of the main reasons we withdraw from emotional confrontations is that we are being overwhelmed emotionally. Research shows that the male cardiovascular and nervous systems are more reactive than those of females. They are also slower to recover from stress after an emotional encounter. This is not true for all men and women. In fact, Carlin seems to be more reactive than I am. But generally men are more reactive than women.

Since strong emotion generally takes a greater toll on the male cardiovascular and nervous systems, it isn't surprising that we tend to avoid emotional confrontations. It isn't that we don't care, as some women fear, but that we are too emotionally overwhelmed to express our feelings.

You can learn to listen without being overwhelmed by telling your partner that you need to listen a little at a time. If you start to become flooded, you need to take a break and come back when you have had a chance to let your nervous system return to normal.

When you start feeling like your partner is always causing problems, you need to remember these biological differences. A woman, who is constitutionally better able to handle stress, more often brings up sensitive issues. A man, who is not as able to handle it, will attempt to avoid getting into the subject.

Women aren't always picking on us and men aren't always withdrawing. The differences come from our evolutionary past, when our differences were necessary. Understanding these patterns and realizing that no one is to blame for these differences, or for the difficulties that arise, can help us to love and appreciate each other. We can communicate with more respect for the unique and wonderful differences that make relationships so interesting.

8. If you want your relationship to be healthier, focus on what you want, not what you don't want.

So many times when we are in pain in our relationship we recite a litany of things that we don't like: I don't like the way I'm being treated. I don't like the way she talks back to me. I don't like the way she looks. I don't like our sex life. Somehow we have the notion that if we can get all the negative things out in the open, things will magically improve.

They usually don't. After working with many people for many years, I have found that what we focus on expands. So when someone comes to me for help and starts telling me all the things that are wrong, the first question I ask is "What would you like instead?"

You don't like the way you are being treated? Great. How would you like to be treated? The answer is usually something like with more respect, kindness, and appreciation. You aren't happy with your sex life? How would you like it to be? More passionate, more frequent, more fun? Moving in a positive direction is much more helpful than trying *not* to move in a negative direction.

I'm not talking about simply thinking positive thoughts and hoping you will get everything you want. You still have to work for the good things in your relationship. But focusing on what you want keeps you looking for solutions, rather than problems. It keeps you wanting to find better ways to expand your love, rather than more reasons to be afraid.

9. Chronic relationship pain needs attention from a specialist. Find one.

With the best of intentions to deal with pain as it arises, many couples find it has become imbedded in the relationship. Men are particularly good at ignoring pain and allowing it to settle in.

It's not surprising that many of us do not respond to acute pain. Pain that is not understood and dealt with becomes chronic. Some of us have become so used to the pain that we don't even notice it anymore.

It's not unusual for me to have a man come into my office and tell me his wife has just left him or is on the verge of leaving. He often looks stunned and confused. He'll tell me he thought they had a pretty good marriage and had no idea she was so unhappy. He talks as if he were completely blindsided. If I get a chance to talk to the woman, she will often tell me that she has been telling him for years that she was in pain and that their relationship was in trouble, but he refused to listen.

Most of us recognize that pains in the chest that radiate down an arm, accompanied by nausea, are signs that we need to see a doctor immediately. These are usually the signs of a problem that has gone on for a long time. Most of us wouldn't try to treat the problem ourselves. We would seek help from a specialist, at least to get a complete evaluation.

However, I do know a man who had all these signs of an imminent heart attack, but kept taking antacids for his "stomach pain" until his wife literally dragged him into the car and took him to the emergency room. After the surgery the doctors told her she had saved his life.

For those of us who have ignored the problem signs our body has been sending us for many years, a heart attack may be the wake-up call that starts us on the path of wellness. For those of us who have ignored the signs of a troubled relationship for years, the wake-up call is often one person leaving, or being on the brink of leaving, the relationship. Sometimes it's the man who says, "I've just got to get out." Sometimes it's the woman who can't take it anymore.

Don't wait until you have a heart attack to get yourself physically healthy, and don't wait until one of you leaves the marriage before you see a relationship specialist. A lot has changed over the years since I began practicing. There is much less stigma about seeing a counselor, and there are many more options to choose from.

There are social workers, marriage and family counselors, psychologists, and psychiatrists. Each specialty offers something a bit different. The key is to find someone you both can work with. Don't be afraid to interview a few before you make your decision.

10. Relationship problems take time to develop and need time to repair, so be patient.

Most of us are action oriented and want quick results. If our car needs repair we expect to go in, tell the mechanic what we think is wrong, drop it off, and pick it up in a few hours. Many of us look at counseling the same way. For many of us, sitting in front of a therapist is a foreign experience. It's almost as though we are hoping we can just drop our relationship off, as we do our suits at the cleaners, and come back in a few days to have them cleaned and pressed and good as new.

Without being aware of it, we often want the therapist to quickly diagnose the problem, fix us, and get our relationship back on the road and running well again. Unfortunately—or fortunately, depending on how you look at it—our relationships are much more complex than our cars or our suits. Fixing them takes more time and active participation from us.

Most of us don't want to acknowledge there is a problem in our relationships. Most of us don't want to come and see a therapist. Most of us want to get it over with as soon as possible. Most of us want to leave after attending one or two sessions. When I went to therapy, I had to remind myself again and again to remember the reason I had come. I wanted my marriage to heal. I wanted to have a relationship that was fun, loving, and playful as it once had been. I wanted to care and feel cared for. I wanted to be together as we grew older.

If you come for help, stay for help. Resist your temptation to get discouraged, drop out, and try something else. You are important. Your relationship is important. Do what it takes to get all the help you need to heal. You will be glad you did.

ACTION OPTION

Decide to Improve Your Relationship

Sit with your partner and read the 10 ways for improving your relationship listed above. Talk about each one and imagine how it might help your relationship. Pick one that you are both willing to try over the next two weeks. Take action. Evaluate the results and see how things change.

PART VI

The Eight-Week Men Alive Health Challenge

CHAPTER 17

Healthier Than You've Ever Been

Masculinity is not something given to you, something you're born with, but something you gain. . . . And you gain it by winning small battles with honor.

—Norman Mailer

I'M LOOKING FOR a group of you who are ready to advance your health in significant ways. I'm sure there are a lot of men who were told they needed my book and never looked at it. Others looked at it, but never bought it. Some bought it, but it sits buried under papers with other things they committed to doing for the New Year.

I know there are some of you who bought the book and have read some, but became busy with life's many demands. Others have read it through, but haven't taken any of the action options. I know how it is; change isn't easy. There are some of you, however, who have taken action or are ready to take action and want to move on to the next challenge. If you are one of those men, I want to talk to you.

Here's what I've learned over the years about men's health in the second half of life. There is one basic truth. We either go downhill and deteriorate, or we move up onto a new mountain that is different, but every bit as wonderful, as the first. In fact, for many of us, the second half is even *better* than the first. Since turning 40 I have had less stress and illness than in the years before. I know that if I follow the directions in this book, which I fully intend to continue doing, I can be even healthier at 70 than I am at 57.

How can that be? I'll tell you what it's been like for me. In my early years I never thought much about taking care of my health. It was just something I assumed would take care of itself. If something broke, I got it fixed and assumed it would be as good as new. I know that if I'd taken that attitude toward my new car, it wouldn't be an old car now; it would have died long ago.

The truth is, I made it this far because I had good genes from my ancestors and a little blind luck that helped me avoid the worst mistakes. But now that I know what is possible, I've become an active agent in my own health. Now that I have the tools to *really* take care of myself, I fully intend to keep becoming healthier as I age. As more and more answers become available from the Human Genome Project and other research that is breaking new ground in our understanding of health, I intend to be at the front of the line to get the information and put it into practice in my own life.

Here's another thing I've learned: The mind has a tremendous effect on our body functions. Some scientists believe that the mind has the *most* effect and that if we keep it focused on health, the body will follow. That's an exciting thought to me. Our minds can remain forever young and acquire more and more wisdom as the years go by.

So here's the deal. I'm looking for men who have the guts, the stamina, and the will to try the full program for eight weeks. If it doesn't work for you, fine. There are many other good programs you can try. However, if it does work, I want you to make a commitment to yourself, to me, and to one other person to make this a part of your life forever.

I don't expect that your health will be turned around in eight weeks. You won't go from a "98-pound health weakling" to a "165-pound health powerhouse," to paraphrase the ads we grew up with from Charles Atlas.

I do expect that your life will change dramatically. As I will show you later in this chapter, all the aspects of health are related and feed each other. Even getting a feel of having all the parts work together will give you the experience of what a healthy life can really be.

Living a healthy, joyful, and passionate life requires continued practice. But what else would you rather do with your life? Do you want it to be unhealthy, joyless, and dull? Remember, there are only two directions you can move in the second half of life. On any given day, week, month, or year you are moving toward either health or disease. You can't go both directions at once. The choice is up to you. The challenge is ahead.

There's something else I need to tell you. Successfully completing the challenge is not for you alone. Remember in our younger days that we used to play the game king of the mountain? There were many variations, but they all had a similar form. There was some obstacle that confronted us and our buddies. Each of us would strive to be the first one to the top and, once there, to keep anyone else from taking our position. The one who remained on top, and kept the others off, won the game.

For many of us the game didn't end in childhood. We played the game in our personal lives, competing with our friends for position and status. We played the game in our work lives, competing with our fellow workers for a place at the top.

If you still want to play that game, by all means do so. But *this* challenge is not for you alone. If you undertake this challenge you will be doing it for your family. Whether you are aware of it or not, they watch your health habits and are influenced either positively or negatively by them.

If you undertake this challenge you will be doing it for younger males. Young men are killing others and dying in the streets. They are committing suicide. They are doing drugs and bingeing on alcohol. They wander through life without direction or desire. There are many reasons for this, but one of the primary reasons is that they don't see older males who give them hope for the future.

If all they see are men over 40 going downhill, there is little that motivates them to look ahead. It isn't surprising that so many of our young men live with the belief that they should grab what they can now, even if it means putting their lives on the line. If you accept this challenge you will be doing it to support them as well.

They may act hostile or indifferent and tell us that we are "old men" with nothing to tell them. Don't believe it. They act with bluster because they have been let down and disappointed so many times. Believe me, they are watching us. They see how we look, how we walk, and whether we are happy or sad, healthy or sick. They need us to model the truth that getting older is a good thing.

Finally, if you accept this challenge you will be doing it for other men. There's probably no group of people that influences us more than the men around us. If all our buddies are putting on weight, becoming depressed, or being inactive, it is a lot easier for us to follow in their footsteps. On the other hand, when we are surrounded by guys who are committed to their own health, it motivates us to do the same.

One of the motivations for me in writing this book comes from the men I know who have gone downhill after 40. Some of them have died, leaving family and friends to carry on without them. I know that if more of us were healthy, fewer men would get sick and die. For every man we influence by simply living healthier lives, there is a ripple effect. He will influence his wife, his sons and daughters, his parents, his friends, and men he doesn't even know.

So are you with me? I know some of you guys are going to complete the challenge in eight weeks. You are the ones I want to hear from first. I want to hear about your experiences. What worked for you and what didn't? What lessons you have learned that might help families, young males, or other men?

Others among you may take more time. There's nothing sacred about doing this program in exactly eight weeks. The important thing is that *if* you commit to doing it, you do it. Remember the time when a man's word was his bond? If we said we would do something, we didn't need a contract to take to court if we failed. That's the kind of relationship we have developed in my men's group. That's the kind of relationship I expect with you.

I know it may take 10 weeks or 10 months or 10 years to hear from some of you. Whatever time it takes, I want to know how you are doing. There is no way we can fail if we keep at it. You can count on me to keep playing my part. I will be here in 10 years and likely many more years in the future. At the end of this chapter you will get the graduation certificate. I will look forward to hearing from you.

Before we begin any serious challenge we need to get ready. I hope what you've read in the book so far has gotten you motivated. However, there is a major drawback in writing a book that I need to discuss with you now.

When writing a book, an author is forced to put complex ideas into easy-to-assimilate bites that a reader can understand and use. Each of the chapters is my attempt to give you a piece of the puzzle that is men's health. Yet in the very act of simplifying we are in danger of losing some of the truth. Focusing separate chapters on the hormonal, physical, nutritional, psychological, interpersonal, and spiritual aspects of men's health implies that these are unique entities in a man's life.

The truth is that all aspects of men's health are highly interdependent. When we change one we change all the others. For instance, we know that when a man feels strong and self-confident his testosterone level goes up, and when a man's testosterone levels are raised his confidence and self-esteem increases. Physical exercise can change our hormonal balance as well as the way we feel and even how we relate to our wives.

The eight-week health challenge will involve combining the separate aspects of health into a comprehensive lifestyle. That can seem like a formidable task. The good news is that by changing any one thing in a healthier direction, you change all the others. So as a warm-up for the challenge I want to give you some examples of the important interrelationships that we have found.

Mind/Emotion/Body/Spirit All Work Together

Exercise and Depression

Research studies have shown for some time that exercise can help manage depression, but new evidence indicates that regular workouts may help soothe a sad psyche as effectively as antidepressants. Researchers at Duke University tested people with major depression and found that a moderate exercise program (30 minutes three times per week) reduced depression as much as medication.

The medications produced results more quickly, but after 16 weeks, the exercise effect caught up, according to the study. Exercise causes the brain to produce serotonin, a neurotransmitter that can reduce depression. In addition to giving certain brain chemicals a boost, working out may enhance your body image and may impart a sense of accomplishment, mastery, and pride.

Weight and Stress

Studies show that chronic stress may lead to more body fat around the middle due to elevated levels of the stress hormone cortisol. If dieting and exercising haven't whittled your ab flab, try adding a relaxation component to your routine, such as daily meditation, yoga, or other stress-reducing activities.

Walking and Mental Agility

In one recent study, walking for 45 minutes three days a week significantly improved the concentration and reaction times of seniors, due to an increased supply of oxygen to areas of the brain controlling those processes.

Active Mind/Body and Alzheimer's Disease

At one of the American Academy of Neurology's annual meetings, a long-term study reported that people who had the greatest involvement in mental and physical activities in their middle years were one-third less likely to develop Alzheimer's disease later in life.

Social Ties and Long Life

In a large 12-year study of older Americans, social activity—traveling, participating in group activities, going out to movies, or attending sporting events—lowered mortality almost as much as physical activity did.

Optimism and Health

Optimism has been linked to better immune function, lowered levels of stress-related chemicals, and longer life—all good reasons to look on the bright side.

Marriage and Longevity

A large international study followed more than 3,300 middle-aged men for a decade. In the end, unmarried guys were 70 percent more likely to be dead than married men. They were more than twice as likely to die of a heart attack.

Sex, Love, and an Amazing Hormone Most of Us Don't Know About (Hint: It Isn't Testosterone)

Scientists are saying they may have discovered the relationship hormone. That's right, a hormone that controls how well we bond to others, especially in romantic relationships. This hormone is known to many women because it is essential for childbirth and nursing, but it's unknown to most men.

The hormone is released by the pituitary gland of men and women during sexual excitement. Its presence also seems important in maintaining a loving connection with our partners. The scientists conclude, "We're not there yet, but this research suggests this underrated hormone may play a key role in keeping couples together."

What is it? Oxytocin. Never heard of it before? Well, join the club. That's what's so exciting about being a man on the journey of total health—physical, emotional, hormonal, nutritional, social, sexual, and spiritual. We discover new things that we can use to enhance our healthy lives.

Are You Ready for the Challenge?

Now that you have a greater idea of the ways all these health practices are related, we will put it all together. I am going to suggest an order to the challenge. If you would like to do the eight weeks in a different order, feel free to make that choice. The important thing is that you complete the following eight steps:

1. Get physical
2. Eat well
3. Expand your mind
4. Work with your emotions
5. Confront your calling
6. Deal with the Woman
7. Deepen your intimacy
8. Tune into your hormones

Remember, the order has nothing to do with the importance of each. They are all important. For a complete health challenge, you need to experience them all. I'm sure someone else might put them in a different order. I might even put them in a different order if I did them a week earlier or a week later.

You will start with the first item—get physical—in week number one. In week number two you will continue doing something physical from week one while you begin to change the way you eat. In week three you will continue doing something physical while eating in a new way, and at the same time you will work to expand your mind. You will continue adding items until in the eighth week you will be doing something from all eight categories.

If this seems like trying to juggle eight balls at once, it only seems that way when you read it. When you actually *do* it, you'll find it's not so difficult.

But I do want to remind you. The challenge ahead is not easy. It will take your very best efforts. It may be the most difficult eight weeks in your life. It may also be the most valuable and health producing. If you're not ready yet, this is the time to stop. If you're ready to go, let's get started. Here's something I have learned that will help us succeed at this challenge (and any others we may attempt in the future): *It's hard by the yard, but a cinch by the inch.*

I don't know if you are anything like me, but I've taken on many challenges in my life. I have to admit I've failed at more than I've succeeded at. The ones that seem the most difficult are the personal life-change challenges I've made over the years. I think back on the times I committed to spending more time with my kids, being more understanding with my wife, changing patterns at work so they would be less stressful, exercising more, losing weight.

I start off like a ball of fire. I'm excited, motivated, and focused. I'm like a sprinter coming out of the blocks to run a race. I usually do quite well for a few weeks or a few months. But then I slide back into old habits and forget about my commitments, or I vow to try it again later when my life is less stressful. Does this sound familiar to you?

Over the years I've come to realize that there is another way. I learned that everything doesn't have to be do or die, black or white, on or off, full speed ahead, or dead in the water. I remembered an experiment we did in our high school biology class. As these kinds of experiments often did, this one involved a frog. This was before the time that we realized that animals also have rights.

In the first part of the experiment, we tested the hypothesis that if we tossed the frog into boiling water, he would feel the change immediately, react to the danger, and jump out immediately. Sure enough, that's what the frog did.

In the second part of the experiment, we tested the hypothesis that if we put the frog into cold water and slowly turned the heat up, he wouldn't notice the change, would feel OK until the heat was harmful, and would die before jumping out. Sure enough, the frog never jumped out and surely would have died if we compassionate students hadn't scooped him out in time.

This concept is known scientifically as the *law of least-noted difference.* It tells us that small changes can go unnoticed and hence can build into big changes without people noticing. This law works against us as we engage in small unhealthy acts that go unnoticed until they get big. Our weight creeps up a pound at a time until we look in the mirror one day or see a picture of ourselves with our guts hanging over our belts, and we can't believe we are looking at us.

A similar thing happens with our physical activity and other aspects of our life. Little by little, one small step at a time, we move away from healthy habits. Sometimes it's the heart attack that wakes us up. Sometimes it's the realization that we can't play ball with our children or grandchildren because we are so out of shape.

However, the same process of small change that started us on the road away from health can be used to move in a healthy direction. Simply stated, taking small steps consistently can be done without feeling that we are working at it. Small changes are a lot easier to make and sustain than large changes.

The eight-week health challenge is built on this idea. We will be taking small steps, moving ahead an inch at a time. But, as you will see, these small steps will quickly build on themselves and support us in taking other small steps. The result will be that you will finish the challenge much easier than you thought possible. You will also find that you can keep going to maintain a healthy lifestyle throughout the years.

Are you ready to rumble? Good. The first thing you need to do is to get a notebook. Title it "My Eight-Week Men Alive Health Challenge." Put your name at the top and the date you begin.

Week One: Get More Physical

To begin, I want you to write down all the physical activities you do and how often you do them. This should include everything from walking up the stairs of your apartment to exercising—three times a week is good—at the gym. This will be your baseline level of activity.

Next, I want you to inch ahead one step. There is a tendency in most of us to want to do too much too fast. "Hey, this is easy," you think. "I can handle this. I'll do a little more and get there faster." Don't do it. Going a little faster now will catch up to you at the end.

Think of yourself as a long-distance runner instead of a sprinter. To have what it takes to finish strongly at the end, you have to discipline yourself at the beginning not to go out too fast. Remember, this is an eight-week challenge. Whatever you do this week you will continue doing every week for the next seven weeks.

Now look over your level of activity and think of increasing it a small amount. Think in terms of no more than 10 percent. If you walk a half hour twice a week, increase it to 33 minutes instead of 30. If you exercise hard at the gym, add a little bit of flexibility exercises to your routine. If you need other ideas or motivation, refer to chapter 9, which deals with physical health.

Write down what you have decided to do. At the end of the week, evaluate your results. If you did what you said, make a check by the agreement and add the date. If you didn't do what you said, think about the reasons and start again next week.

Week Two: Eat Well, Don't Eat Sick

You're doing great. Keep doing what you're doing and add in good food.

There is a joke about the guy at the bar extolling the virtues of Irish coffee. "Yeah," he says, "it's got your four basic food groups: sugar, fat, caffeine, and alcohol." There's a great deal of wisdom in this statement, even though it is obviously false.

It's not surprising that so many of us have a difficult time eating well. We are surrounded by foods that are not only unhealthy, but seem to be ones that we so easily crave. When we reflect on our food habits, our bodies seem to work against us. We often wonder, if fruits and vegetables are so good for us, why don't we have a hunger for citrus fruits, carrots, and broccoli instead of chocolate cake, Big Macs, and Häagen Dazs ice cream? Chapter 7 tells you why.

This week's challenge is very simple. We will eat fewer of the foods our body craves and more foods that our body needs for health. Remember, I said this is simple. I didn't say it would be easy.

Make a list of foods you crave. My list would look like this: cookies, cakes, pastries, pies, red meat, french fries, popcorn with butter at the movies, peanut butter, jams and jellies.

Make a list of fruits and vegetables you like, but find you don't eat enough. For me, I would include corn, string beans, carrots, tomatoes, asparagus, beets, berries, apples, oranges, pears, and plums.

Take two foods from the "I crave" list that you like a lot and eat often and eliminate them during this week. Keep track through the week of how easy or difficult it is and how you feel when you see these foods advertised or see someone else eating them.

Take two foods from the "healthy" list, one fruit and one vegetable that you like but don't eat very often, and increase them in your diet this week. Remember, there are a lot of healthy foods that we enjoy. However, just as our muscles shrink if we don't use them, our enjoyment of a wide range of good foods diminishes if we neglect eating them. Take note of how you feel throughout the week.

There are a few things I have found to be helpful for this challenge and for eating well in general.

1. If we always eat what we "like" or what "tastes good," we will overeat fats, refined carbohydrates, and sugars.
2. If we eat what we know is good for us, our taste buds will become accustomed to those foods, and we will find them more and more enjoyable to eat.
3. Eating poorly and eating fast go together. Try to avoid fast-food places and take time to enjoy your meals.
4. For many of us, some foods are like drugs: We need to eliminate them from our diet altogether. For me, trying to eat one chocolate chip cookie is like an alcoholic trying to have just one drink.
5. Eating well and *not* eating the unhealthy foods we crave is a lifelong process. Remember, the food and beverage industries are working against us. It will take courage, perseverance, and stamina to come out on top. You will be glad you did. So will your family and friends.

Week Three: Expand Your Mind

Remember, as you begin week three you will continue to do some physical activity from week one and the nutritional steps from week two. I think you will see, as the weeks continue, the importance of taking small steps rather than big ones.

I used to think that all the talk about "mind over matter, what you believe you can achieve," was just a lot of hokum. I thought that if you wanted to achieve anything in life, no amount of thinking was going to make it happen. Over the years I've come to recognize that I was both right and wrong.

It's true that we can't *just* think ourselves into health. But I was wrong in not understanding the power of the mind, not only in achieving our goals in life but in actually changing the biochemistry of the body. There are hundreds of scientific studies now that clearly demonstrate that the mind can influence the body.

It's time for you to expand your mind. I want you to think about some part of your body that has been causing you some pain. It could be an old injury from school, a pulled muscle you got yesterday, or anything in your body that hurts. In your notebook, write down the part of your body and the specific kind and level of discomfort you feel.

Your entry would look something like this.:

> Neck: Stiff most of the time. Dull, aching pain on the left side when I turn my neck.

Now I want you find a place where you won't be disturbed. Sit quietly. Close your eyes. Picture your neck surrounded by light. In your mind's eye imagine that it is healthy, fully movable without any discomfort. Continue to sit with this image in your mind for 60 seconds. You can put on a timer or judge when you think a minute has passed.

That's it—a minute a day to expand your mind. We won't worry whether you believe it or see results immediately. Just do it. At the end of the week, write down what you've completed from week one and week two. Once you've completed both, move on to the next week's challenge.

Remember, some of the week's activities will be more difficult for some of us than others. If you forget to do it, or don't do your exercise from the previous week, it doesn't mean you are a failure. It just means you need more work at that level, and you should restart at that level.

Week Four: Work Your Emotions

As you work this week, remember to continue practicing expanding your mind, eating well, and doing something physical.

Emotions are often difficult areas of expression for us. When we are asked, "How do you feel?" our answer is often a shrug of the shoulders or a curt "I don't know." I have found that there are three communication barriers that lie hidden beneath our response. Number one, we don't know if we are feeling emotions. Number two, we are feeling something, but we don't know what words to use to describe it. Number three, we've got the words, but we are afraid to let the other person know how we are feeling.

Our work this week will be focused on all three levels. The first thing we need to know about emotions is that they are expressed first as body sensations. Think about a time when you were very angry. Do you remember some of the things going on in your body? You may have found yourself breathing more shallowly and quickly. You may have noticed your jaw clenching or your heart beating faster. Hurt, fear, guilt, shame, and joy have their own body sensations.

Once we've identified that something is going on in our body that has the sensation of an emotion, we need to learn how to name it. Learning to name our emotions is like learning vocabulary. The more we learn, the better able we are to communicate more subtle aspects of how we are feeling. We'll start with expressing four basic feelings: anger, hurt, fear, and joy.

When we have a "feeling vocabulary" we can practice expressing our feelings in situations that we have avoided in the past. Maybe it's telling your wife that you felt hurt by something she said. It could be telling a friend how much you enjoy being with him.

For this week's challenge, you will pick one of the three levels to practice. Some of us need practice being aware of feeling sensations in our bodies. Others need practice putting names to what we are feeling. The rest of us need help expressing feelings when we are with others.

Here's the challenge for those of you in the first group. During the week, notice what goes on in your body when you are in situations that trigger emotion. Write down what you notice. Your log might look like this:

Monday: Kids fighting in living room. I noticed tension in my neck.

Wednesday: Pressure at work to complete project. I noticed my stomach rumbling.

For those of you in the second group, the challenge is to name all four emotions: anger, hurt, fear, and joy. Your log might look like this:

> Monday: Back to the office. Report I needed had not been done. I felt angry.
> Wednesday: My wife made a comment about my weight. I felt hurt by what she said and how she said it.
> Thursday: I went to visit my father who has been ill. I felt afraid that he might die soon.
> Saturday: Our whole family got together for a picnic. I felt joyful thinking that we were together and healthy.

Do your best to find instances where you have felt all four feelings. Most of us find that we are better at noticing some feelings than others. Some of us may be better at anger, while others may find we feel hurt more often. If you find yourself having difficulty tuning into some emotions, don't worry. With practice, you will be able to express all four and many more.

The third group has a vocabulary for expressing feelings but is reluctant to engage with others. Particularly when talking to women, we may feel afraid that in sharing our feelings it may trigger feelings in our partners that might overwhelm us. The challenge here is to practice saying how you feel to another person and noticing the fear or resistance that may come up as you do it. You can practice expressing how you feel towards your wife, boss, children, or a friend.

Pick one person you'd like to engage. Look for times when you are feeling one of the four feelings. Tell them how you feel. Your log may look like this:

> Monday: I told my wife, Mary, how joyful I felt when she held me.
> Tuesday: I told my son I was angry when he dented the car.

Remember that feelings register in your body. There is a difference between feeling a feeling and thinking about a feeling. When you are feeling hurt, your body may slump and contract, your chest may narrow, and your shoulders may turn in. You may feel tears welling up in your eyes and your throat may constrict. When you are thinking about feeling hurt, you are in your head, not your body. You may be in a situation you think should make you feel a certain way, but you really don't feel it.

To really feel, we need to open ourselves and become vulnerable. We can't feel and remain safe and protected at the same time. There are clearly many situations where we should keep our feelings to ourselves. The purpose of this challenge isn't to teach us how to wear our feelings on our sleeves; it's to allow us to be able to share our feelings when we are with someone we trust. Feelings are not right or wrong. They just are.

Week Five: Heed Your Spiritual Calling

Remember to continue activities from the previous weeks as you engage the new activity for this week.

Our calling is our spiritual gift to ourselves and others in the second half of life. It connects us to the spiritual dimension of our lives. It's what keeps our juices flowing and provides the passion for our continued growth as we age. Those of us who are living our calling never contemplate retiring from work. For me it would be as unthinkable as retiring from eating good food, enjoying good music, or having good sex. Those of us who think about retirement usually are tired of doing what we've been doing for so many years. We are stressed out, run down, and need a rest. However, we don't need to sit in the sun and play golf all day; we need to find and practice our calling.

The challenge for this week is to deepen this commitment. Here are a number of exercises you can do to help you find or express more fully your work in the second half of life.

In your notebook, write a one-page obituary of your life if you died today. Think about the highlights of your life. What are the things that would be memorable about your life? What things would be missing?

Write another obituary that would highlight your life if you lived another 40 years. Think about what you would do that you haven't done so far. Where would you give more of your time, your support, and your love?

Think of one thing you know that if everyone else in the world knew and practiced, the world would be a better place. Write a page on what that would be and what you might do to express this more in your own life.

One of the reasons I have described this work as our calling is because it does call to us. It is quiet at first, but if we don't listen it gets louder. If we deny or ignore the call we begin to sicken inside. When we heed the call our lives expand greatly.

Week Six: Explore Your Feelings toward the Woman

Continue doing the activities from each of the previous five weeks as you work on week six.

Most of us grew up with a lot of confusing messages about women. We heard about the battle of the sexes. We wondered with Professor Henry Higgins, in the play *My Fair Lady,* "Why can't a woman be more like a man?" From the time we were young boys, I believe, deep in our psyches, we viewed females as mysterious, desirable, and dangerous.

In order to come to peace with females generally, or the archetypal Woman as I call her, we have to confront these three aspects of our beliefs and feelings. This is the focus of the week-six challenge.

Think about the *mystery* of the Woman. What things come to mind? Write them down. It is only the Woman who can carry new life in her body, go through the dangerous birth process, and nurture a baby from her own breasts. How does that make you feel? Let those feelings expand and deepen. Write them down.

Think about our *desire* for the Woman. What can she give that we feel we can't get anywhere else? Think about our hunger for nurturing, a soft caress, the feel of her body, her breasts, her vagina, her womanly smell. Look deeply. How do you feel? Record your thoughts and feelings.

Think about our *fear* of the Woman. I remember that as a boy of 10 or 11, I was warned by an older boy who seemed to be wise in the ways of women. "Be careful if you ever put your thing inside her," he told me, his tone authoritative and conspiratorial. "If she crosses her legs you won't be able to get out." When I looked skeptical he reminded me of dogs we'd seen who seemed to be stuck together.

Though we can laugh at our youthful ignorance, the fears of the Woman are real. In every culture throughout the world there are artistic depictions of what a woman can do to a man.

I believe there are universal fears that we all have about the potential of the Woman to overwhelm and destroy us. What are yours? Let your mind go, and remember times when the fears ran deep. What comes to mind? If you have trouble remembering, take a break. Be open. Memories will emerge. Write down whatever comes up for you.

Think about relationships you've had with specific women in your life. How have your feelings of mystery, desire, and fear of the Woman affected your relationships? Write down your thoughts and feelings.

Week Seven: Develop and Deepen Intimacy

Keep going. You're almost there now. Continue your prior six weekly practices as you explore issues of intimacy.

We've all had moments of intimacy. Most of us would like to have more. We have experienced intimate relationships that became dulled over time and intimate relations that drifted away. In this challenge we will be exploring what has gone right in our world and what has gone wrong.

Begin by writing the names of all the people you have had an intimate relationship with, or had reason to expect that you would have an intimate relationship. Include your mother and father and any other people who played a part in your upbringing. If you can't remember someone's name, make one up for this challenge. Once you have listed them in your journal, rate each relationship from 1 to 10—1 being the absolute minimal degree of intimacy and 10 being the most intimate relationship you could imagine.

For the purposes of the challenge we will assume that for each relationship, including the ones with your parents, you did some things that enhanced intimacy and some things that blocked intimacy.

Look over the names and think about each relationship. First focus on the things you did that blocked intimacy. Write them down in your journal. My things would look like this:

My irritability and periodic rages.
Hiding behind my work.
Emotional withdrawal.
Refusing to seek professional help when needed.
Fear of telling the truth about my unhappiness.
Demands for affection and intimacy.

Now look over your relationships again and focus on the things you did that enhanced intimacy. What are the things you have done that you think helped bring about greater intimacy, regardless of whether it was reciprocated by the other person? Write your responses in your journal. My things look like this:

I'm loyal.
I listen well.
I'm caring.
I'm tenacious and will keep trying to make things right.
I am kind.

Now think of the most important relationship you have currently. What are your intimacy-enhancing qualities that would help improve your relationship? What are your intimacy-blocking qualities? During this week, bring more of the positive qualities into your relationship and remove any of the intimacy-blocking qualities that you observe in yourself.

As I've said before, developing and sustaining an intimate relationship is the graduate school of life. If our primary task on the planet is to learn how to love, intimate relationships are the place to do it. Nothing is more difficult, and nothing is more rewarding.

Week 8: Tune into Your Hormones

This is it. One more week and you've made it. Keep your seven weekly practices going as you take a closer look at your hormones.

You are in the homestretch when you've gotten this far in the challenge. For me, this is one of the most interesting and fun parts of the challenge because I knew so little about hormones when I began this project. If you are like me, understanding your hormones isn't on the top of your list of "have-to-know" items.

This week's challenge involves getting to know more about hormones in general and getting to know more about *our* hormones in particular.

Your first task is to reread the chapter on hormones earlier in the book. Take a half hour to write about your thoughts, feelings, and ideas after reviewing chapter 3.

Next, make an appointment with your doctor to have your testosterone levels checked. As you know, our testosterone levels drop as we age. Since there is a great deal of variation of normal levels in men, it is a good idea to know what *your* level is so that you can see how it changes over the years.

While you are at the doctor's office, ask to have your prostate checked if you haven't had it done recently. You'll be glad you did.

I don't expect you to have seen the doctor, had the tests, and gotten the results during the challenge. To complete the challenge you only need to make the appointment, ask for the tests, and commit to following through.

When you finish the challenge there are some additional things I want you to do.

1. Give yourself a round of applause and a pat on the back. You've done something great for yourself and others.

2. Write in your journal about how the challenge was for you. What did you find easy? What was difficult? What did you learn about yourself that surprised you? What do you need to do to incorporate what you've learned into your life? If you'd like, send your thoughts to me. I'd very much like to hear about your experiences so I can incorporate them into my continuing work with men.

3. Pass on what you've learned to someone else. Talk to your son, share your experience with a young man at work, tell a buddy.

4. Fill out your graduation certificate.

5. If you'd like to be listed on our honor roll and receive updates on living long and well, send your information to me. Be sure and send your name and address, particularly your e-mail address, and the date you completed the challenge.

Jed Diamond
E-mail: Jed@menalive.com

THE EIGHT-WEEK MEN'S HEALTH CHALLENGE
GRADUATION CERTIFICATE

This is to certify that ______________________________
has completed the challenge on this ____day of _________, 20__.

He agrees to continue his health practices and be a role model for his family, younger males, and the other men and women in his life.

Jed Diamond, Director, MenAlive
www.MenAlive.com

MEN'S HEALTH RESOURCES

This is a very small portion of all that is available. I have found that most people have access to a computer and so can access health sites on the Web. These are the sites that I use the most and have found to be particularly helpful. If you find others you think should be added, please let me know.

Androc Corporation
Dedicated to enriching and prolonging the quality of life for the aging male through proactive preventative medicine, timely and appropriate medical intervention, and the development and application of research and education.
Web address: *http://www.androc.com*

E-Medicine Andro Screen Center
This is an important site created by Malcolm Carruthers, M.D., one of the world's experts on male menopause. It offers information on testosterone replacement therapy (TRT) and the treatment of male menopause, or andropause.
Web address: *http://www.goldcrossmedical.com*

Everyman
A wonderful journal featuring general men's issues that is published bimonthly.
Address: P.O. Box 4617, Station E, Ottawa, ON, K1S 5H8 Canada
Phone: 613-832–2284
Web address: *http://www.everyman.org*

Dr. Warren Farrell
Warren has been one of the key leaders in the men's health movement since his first book, *The Liberated Man,* was published in 1975. Here you can learn about his most recent work.
Web address: *http://www.warrenfarrell.com*

Health Central
Dr. Dean Edell, one of the nation's leading experts on health, has developed this site with the consumer in mind. It is easy to access and use and I recommend it highly.
Web address: *http://www.healthcentral.com*

Healthfinder®
This is a free gateway to reliable consumer health and human services information developed by the U.S. Department of Health and Human Services. It has a host of general health information as well as a good section on men's health.
Web address: *http://www.healthfinder.gov*

John Lee (men's issues and feelings)
John Lee has committed 20 years of his life to helping people live richer and fuller lives by teaching them to release the emotions trapped inside their bodies.
Web address: *http://www.flyingboy.com*

Male Health Center
The oldest, and still one of the few centers in the country devoted specifically to men's health. It was started by men's health expert Kenneth Goldberg, M.D.
Web address: *http://www.malehealthcenter.com*

Mankind Project (formerly New Warrior Network)
Men leading lives of integrity and connection to feeling. The group sponsors initiation weekends for men and boys.
Web address: *http://www.mkp.org*
E-mail: moreinfo@mkp.org

Men Alive
Resources on living long and well, men's health, and male menopause, compiled by Jed Diamond.
Web address: *http://www.menalive.com*

Men's Center
Assists men in finding male-positive resources, information, and support. Has links to many other men's centers throughout the country.
Web address: *http://www.themenscenter.com*

Men's Health
An online magazine with a range of resources, games, surveys, quizzes, ask the sex doc, workouts, and more.
Web address: *http://www.menshealth.com*

Men's Health Consulting

A wonderful resource developed by longtime men's health proponent Will Courtenay. MHC is an educational and training firm that promotes better health and wellness in men and boys.

Web address: *http://www.menshealth.org*

Men's Health Network

A national informational and educational organization recognizing men's health as a specific social concern.

Web address: *http://www.menshealthnetwork.org*

Menstuff: The National Men's Resource

Serving men since 1982. A true wealth of information on men, men's issues, and men's health.

Address: Box 800-W, San Anselmo, CA 94979

Web address: *http:// www.menstuff.org*

MenWeb

A wonderful web site with a large number of articles and resources maintained as a labor of love by Bert Hoff, formerly of the Seattle Men's Evolvement Network (M.E.N. Magazine)

Web address: *http://www.vix.com/menmag*

National Organization to Halt the Abuse and Routine Mutilation of Males (NOHARMM)

Men opposed to infant circumcision in defense of children's rights. Raises public awareness about male genital cutting (MGC) practices and increases public understanding of genital integrity as a fundamental human right.

Address: P.O. Box 460795, San Francisco, CA 94146

Phone: 415/826–9351

Web address: *http://www.noharmm.org*

New England Centenarian Study

Based at Beth Israel Deaconess Medical Center and Harvard Medical School, the New England Centenarian Study's mission is to study centenarians (those over 100) who they believe carry the secrets to successful aging and how to delay or even escape diseases associated with aging.

Web address: *http://www.med.harvard.edu/programs/necs*

Sterling Institute of Relationships

Offers weekend initiations and rites of passage for men of all ages. The weekend experience focuses on the unique differences between males and females and how these differences can help create natural and loving relationships.

Web address: *http://www.higherpurpose.com*

Dr. Andrew Weil's Self Healing

A tremendous resource from one of our leading doctors and health advocates. Dr. Weil also has a newsletter that I highly recommend.

Web address: *http://www.drweilselfhealing.com*

SELECTED BIBLIOGRAPHY

Adams, Patch, with Maureen Mylander. *Gesundheit! Bringing Good Health to You, the Medical System, and Society through Physician Service, Complementary Therapies, Humor, and Joy.* Rochester, Vt.: Healing Arts Press, 1993.

Barash, David P., and Judith Eve Lipton. *Making Sense of Sex: How Genes and Gender Influence Our Relationships.* Washington, D.C.: Island Press, 1997.

Barrie, James M. *Peter Pan.* London: Samuel French, 1928.

Blankenhorn, David. *Fatherless America: Confronting Our Most Urgent Social Problem.* New York: Basic Books, 1995.

Bortz, Walter M., II. *Dare to Be 100.* New York: Fireside, 1996.

Campbell, Joseph. *The Power of Myth.* New York: Viking, 1988.

Carnes, Mark C. *Secret Ritual and Manhood in Victorian America.* New Haven, Conn.: Yale University Press, 1989.

Carruthers, Malcolm. *Maximising Manhood: Beating the Male Andropause.* London: HarperCollins, 1997.

Cetron, Marvin, and Owen Davies. *Cheating Death.* New York: St. Martin's, 1998.

Coon, Carlton. *The Hunting People.* London: Jonathan Cape, 1971.

Courtenay, Will H. "Behavioral Factors Associated with Disease, Injury, and Death Among Men: Evidence and Implications for Prevention." *Journal of Men's Studies* 9, no. 1 (2000): pp. 81–142.

Crenshaw, Theresa L. *The Alchemy of Love and Lust.* New York: G. P. Putnam's Sons, 1996.

Crose, Royda. *Why Women Live Longer Than Men.* San Francisco: Jossey-Bass, 1997.

Cutler, Winnifred. *Love Cycles: The Science of Intimacy.* New York: Villard, 1991.

Diamond, Carlin. *Love It, Don't Label It: A Practical Guide for Using Spiritual Principles in Everyday Life.* Willits, Calif.: Fifth Wave Press, 1985.

Diamond, Jed. *The Warrior's Journey Home: Healing Men, Healing the Planet.* Oakland: New Harbinger Publications, 1994.

_______. *Looking for Love in All the Wrong Places: Overcoming Romantic and Sexual Addictions.* New York: G. P. Putnam's Sons, 1988.

_______. *Inside Out: Becoming My Own Man.* Willits, Calif.: Fifth Wave Press, 1983.

Eaton, S. Boyd, Marjorie Shostak, and Melvin Konner. *The Paleolithic Prescription: A Program of Diet and Exercise and a Design for Living.* New York: Harper & Row, 1988.

Edell, Dean. *Eat, Drink and Be Merry.* New York: HarperCollins, 1999.

Faludi, Susan. *Stiffed: The Betrayal of the American Man.* New York: William Morrow, 1999.

Farrell, Warren. *Father and Child Reunion: How to Bring the Dads We Need to the Children We Love.* New York: Jeremy P. Tarcher/Putnam, 2000.

_______. *The Myth of Male Power.* New York: Simon & Schuster, 1993.

_______. *The Liberated Man.* New York: Random House, 1975.

Fisher, Helen. *The First Sex.* New York: Random House, 1999.

Gilligan, James. *Violence: Our Deadly Epidemic and Its Causes.* New York: G. P. Putnam's Sons, 1996.

Gilmore, David. *Manhood in the Making: Cultural Concepts of Masculinity.* New Haven, Conn.: Yale University Press, 1990.

Gittleman, Ann Louise. *Super Nutrition for Men and the Women Who Love Them.* New York: M. Evans, 1996.

Goldberg, Herb. *The Hazards of Being Male: Surviving the Myths of Masculine Privilege.* Plainview, N.Y: Nash Publishing, 1976.

Goldberg, Ken. *When the Man You Love Won't Take Care of His Health.* New York: St. Martin's, 1999.

_______. *How Men Can Live As Long As Women.* Fort Worth: Summit Group, 1993.

Gottman, John. *Why Marriages Succeed or Fail.* New York: Simon & Schuster, 1994.

Gottman, John, and Nan Silver. *The Seven Principles for Making Marriage Work.* New York: Crown, 1999.

Greer, Germaine. *The Change: Women, Aging and the Menopause.* New York: Ballantine, 1991.

Gurian, Michael. *The Wonder of Boys.* New York: G. P. Putnam's Sons, 1996.

Gutmann, David. *Reclaimed Powers.* Evanston, Ill.: Northwestern University Press, 1994.

Hallowell, Edward. *Worry: Controlling It and Using It Wisely.* New York: Pantheon, 1997.

Hill, Aubrey. *The Testosterone Solution.* Rocklin, Calif.: Prima Publishing, 1997.

Hill, Julia Butterfly. *The Legacy of Luna: The Story of a Tree, a Woman, and the Struggle to Save the Redwoods.* New York: HarperCollins, 2000.

Hillman, James. *The Force of Character and the Lasting Life.* New York: Random House, 1999.

_______. *The Soul's Code: In Search of Character and Calling.* New York: Random House, 1996.

Hitchcox, Lee. *Long Life Now.* Berkeley, Calif.: Celestial Arts, 1996.

Jamison, Kay Redfield. *An Unquiet Mind: Memoir of Moods and Madness.* New York: Vintage, 1996.

Janeway, Elizabeth. *Man's World, Woman's Place: A Study in Social Mythology.* New York: Dell, 1971.

Kauth, Bill. *A Circle of Men: For Starting a Men's Group, for Existing Men's Groups.* New York: St. Martin's, 1992.

Keen, Sam. *Fire in the Belly: On Being a Man.* New York: Bantam, 1991.

Kipnis, Aaron, and Elizabeth Herron. *Gender War, Gender Peace: The Quest for Justice between Women and Men.* New York: William Morrow, 1994.

Klatz, Ronald. *Grow Young with HGH.* New York: HarperCollins, 1997.

Lee, Richard B., and Irven De Vore, eds. *Man the Hunter.* Chicago: Aldine, 1968.

Mander, Jerry. *In the Absence of the Sacred: The Failure of Technology and the Survival of the Indian Nations.* San Francisco: Sierra Club Books, 1991.

McDougall, John A., and Mary A. McDougall. *The McDougall Plan.* Piscataway, N.J.: New Century Publishers, 1983.

Ness, Randolph M., and George C. Williams. *Why We Get Sick.* New York: Random House, 1994.

Pearsall, Paul. *Sexual Healing: Using the Power of an Intimate, Loving Relationship to Heal Your Body and Soul.* New York: Crown, 1994.

Perls, Thomas T., and Margery Hutter Silver. *Living to 100.* New York: Basic Books, 1999.

Polenz, Joanna Magda. *The Last Sick Generation.* Tampa: American College of Physician Executives, 2000.

Rako, Susan. *The Hormone of Desire.* New York: Three Rivers Press, 1996.

Real, Terrence. *I Don't Want to Talk About It: Overcoming the Secret Secrecy of Male Depression.* New York: Scribner, 1997.

Regelson, William, and Carol Colman. *The Superhormone Promise: Nature's Antidote to Aging.* New York: Simon & Schuster, 1996.

Ridley, Matt. *The Red Queen: Sex and the Evolution of Human Nature.* New York: Macmillian, 1993.

Ritter, Thomas T. *Say No to Circumcision: 40 Compelling Reasons Why You Should Respect His Birthright and Keep Your Son Whole.* Aptos, Calif. Hourglass Book Publishing, 1992.

Robbins John. *Diet for a New America.* Walpole, N.H.: Stillpoint Publishing, 1987.

Robertson, Joel, with Tom Monte. *Natural Prozac: Learning to Release Your Body's Own Anti-Depressants.* San Francisco: HarperCollins, 1997.

Sahlins, Marshall D. *Stone Age Economics.* Chicago: Aldine Atherton, 1972.

Schenk, Roy U., and John Everingham. *Men Healing Shame: An Anthology.* New York: Springer Publishing, 1995.

Schmookler, Andrew B. *The Parable of the Tribes: The Problem of Power in Social Evolution.* Boston: Houghton Mifflin, 1984.

Shippen, Eugene, and William Fryer. *The Testosterone Syndrome.* New York: M. Evans, 1998.

Somé, Malidoma P. *Of Water and the Spirit: Ritual, Magic, and Initiation in the Life of an African Shaman.* New York: G. P. Putnam's Sons, 1994.

Taylor, George. *Talking with Our Brothers: Creating and Sustaining a Dynamic Men's Group.* Fairfax, Calif.: Men's Community Publishing Project, 1995.

Trungpa, Chögyam. *Shambhala: The Sacred Path of the Warrior.* Boston: Shambhala Publications, 1984.

Weil, Andrew. *Eating Well for Optimum Health.* New York: Random House, 2000.

Weiner, Bernard. *Boy into Man: A Father's Guide to Initiation of Teenage Sons.* San Francisco: Transformation Press, 1992.

Wright, Jonathan V., and Lane Lenard. *Maximize Your Vitality and Potency.* Petaluma, Calif.: Smart Publications, 1999.

INDEX